Your *Clinics* subscription just got better!

W9-CES-191

You can now access the FULL TEXT of this publication online at no additional cost! Activate your online subscription today and receive...

- Full text of all issues from 2002 to the present
- Photographs, tables, illustrations, and references
- Comprehensive search capabilities
- Links to MEDLINE and Elsevier journals

Activate Your Online Access Today!

Plus, you can also sign up for E-alerts of upcoming issues or articles that interest you, and take advantage of exclusive access to bonus features!

To activate your individual online subscription:

1. Visit our website at **www.TheClinics.com**.

2. Click on "Register" at the top of the page, and follow the instructions.

3. To activate your account, you will need your subscriber account number, which you can find on your mailing label (note: the number of digits in your subscriber account number varies from six to ten digits). See the sample below where the subscriber account number has been circled.

This is your subscriber account number

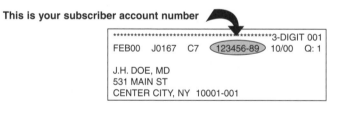

```
******************************************3-DIGIT 001
FEB00   J0167   C7   123456-89   10/00   Q: 1

J.H. DOE, MD
531 MAIN ST
CENTER CITY, NY  10001-001
```

4. That's it! Your online access to the most trusted source for clinical reviews is now available.

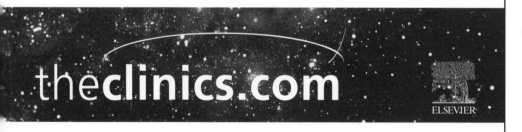

theclinics.com

ELSEVIER

theclinics.com

SURGICAL CLINICS
OF NORTH AMERICA

Laparoscopic Surgery:
Beyond Mere Feasibility

GUEST EDITORS
Nilesh A. Patel, MD
Roberto Bergamaschi, MD, PhD

February 2005 • Volume 85 • Number 1

SAUNDERS

An Imprint of Elsevier, Inc.
PHILADELPHIA   LONDON   TORONTO   MONTREAL   SYDNEY   TOKYO

W.B. SAUNDERS COMPANY
A Division of Elsevier Inc.

The Curtis Center • Independence Square West • Philadelphia, Pennsylvania 19106

http://www.theclinics.com

SURGICAL CLINICS OF NORTH AMERICA   Volume 85, Number 1
February 2005   ISSN 0039–6109
Editor: Catherine Bewick   ISBN 1-4160-2790-4

The ideas and opinions expressed in *The Surgical Clinics of North America* do not necessarily reflect those of the Publisher. The Publisher does not assume any responsibility for any injury and/or damage to persons or property arising out of or related to any use of the material contained in this periodical. The reader is advised to check the appropriate medical literature and the product information currently provided by the manufacturer of each drug to be administered to verify the dosage, the method and duration of administration, or contraindications. It is the responsibility of the treating physician or other health care professional, relying on independent experience and knowledge of the patient, to determine drug dosages and the best treatment for the patient. Mention of any product in this issue should not be construed as endorsement by the contributors, editors, or the Publisher of the product or manufacturers' claims.

Surgical Clinics of North America (ISSN 0039–6109) is published bimonthly by Elsevier; Corporate and editorial Offices: 170 S Independence Mall W 300 E, Philadelphia, PA 19106-3399. Accounting and circulation offices: 6277 Sea Harbor Drive, Orlando, FL 32887-4800. Periodicals postage paid at Orlando, FL 32862, and additional mailing offices. Subscription prices are $190.00 per year for US individuals, $299.00 per year for US institutions, $95.00 per year for US students and residents, $234.00 per year for Canadian individuals, $365.00 per year for Canadian institutions, $250.00 for international individuals, $365.00 for international institutions and $125.00 per year for Canadian and foreign students/residents. To receive student/resident rate, orders must be accompanied by name of affiliated institution, date of term, and the *signature* of program/residency coordinator on institution letterhead. Orders will be billed at individual rate until proof of status is received. Foreign air speed delivery is included in all *Clinics* subscription prices. All prices are subject to change without notice. POSTMASTER: Send address changes to *The Surgical Clinics of North America*, W.B. Saunders Company, Periodicals Fulfillment, Orlando, FL 32887-4800. **Customer Service: 1-800-654-2452 (US). From outside of the US, call 1-407-345-1000.**

The Surgical Clinics of North America is also published in Spanish by McGraw-Hill Interamericana Editores S.A., P.O. Box 5-237 06500 Mexico D.F. Mexico; and in Portuguese by Interlivros Edicoes Ltda., Rua Comandante Coelho 1085, CEP 21250, Rio de Janeiro, Brazil; and in Greek by Paschalidis Medical Publications, Athens Greece.

The Surgical Clinics of North America is covered in *Index Medicus, EMBASE/Excerpta Medica, Current Contents/Clinical Medicine, Current Contents/Life Sciences, Science Citation Index*, and *ISI/BIOMED.*

Printed in the United States of America.

GUEST EDITORS

NILESH A. PATEL, MD, Staff Surgeon, Department of Surgery, Divisions of Bariatric and General Surgery, Allegheny General Hospital, Pittsburgh, Pennsylvania

ROBERTO BERGAMASCHI, MD, PhD, FRCS, FASCRS, FACS, Director, Minimally Invasive Surgery Center; Director, Minimally Invasive Surgery Fellowship Program, Allegheny General Hospital; and Professor of Surgery, Drexel University College of Medicine, Pittsburgh, Pennsylvania

CONTRIBUTORS

ORHAN ALIMOGLU, MD, Department of Surgery, Vakif Teaching Hospital, Istanbul, Turkey

O. AZIZ, BSc (Hons), MBBS, MRCS, Research Fellow, Department of Surgical Oncology and Technology, Imperial College, London, England

SUSAN M. CERA, MD, Clinical Associate, Department of Colorectal Surgery, Cleveland Clinic Florida, Weston, Florida

C.C. CHUNG, FRCSEd (Gen), Minimal Access Surgery Training Centre, Department of Surgery, Pamela Youde Nethersole Eastern Hospital, Hong Kong

WILLIAM S. COBB, MD, Fellow, Carolinas Laparoscopic and Advanced Surgery Program, Carolinas Medical Center, Charlotte, North Carolina

A. DARZI, MD, FRCS, FACS, FRCSI, Professor of Surgery, Department of Surgical Oncology and Technology, Imperial College, London, England

GEORGE A. FIELDING, MBBS, Associate Professor, Department of Surgery, New York University School of Medicine, New York, New York

MICHEL GAGNER, MD, FRCS, FACS, Professor of Surgery; Chief, Division of Bariatric Surgery, Department of Surgery, Joan and Stanford I. Weill Medical College of Cornell University, New York Presbyterian Hospital, New York, New York

B. TODD HENIFORD, MD, Chief, Minimal Access Surgery, Carolinas Laparoscopic and Advanced Surgery Program, Carolinas Medical Center, Charlotte, North Carolina

KENT W. KERCHER, MD, Co-Director, Carolinas Laparoscopic and Advanced Surgery Program, Carolinas Medical Center, Charlotte, North Carolina

IRENA KIRMAN, MD, PhD, Assistant Professor, Department of Surgery, College of Physicians and Surgeons of Columbia University, New York, New York

SEIGO KITANO, MD, FACS, Department of Surgery I, Faculty of Medicine, Oita University, Oita, Japan

S.Y. KWOK, FRCSEd (Gen), Minimal Access Surgery Training Centre, Department of Surgery, Pamela Youde Nethersole Eastern Hospital, Hong Kong

DAVE R. LAL, MD, Acting Instructor and Senior Fellow, Department of Surgery, Center for Videoendoscopic Surgery, University of Washington, Seattle, Washington

M.K.W. LI, FRCS, Minimal Access Surgery Training Centre, Department of Surgery, Pamela Youde Nethersole Eastern Hospital, Hong Kong

RONALD MATTEOTTI, MD, Research Fellow, Laparoscopic Surgery, Department of Surgery, Joan and Stanford I. Weill Medical College of Cornell University, New York Presbyterian Hospital, New York, New York

JEFFREY W. MILSOM, MD, Professor of Surgery, Chief, Section of Colorectal Surgery, New York Presbyterian Hospital, Weill Medical College of Cornell University, New York, New York

BRANT K. OELSCHLAGER, MD, Assistant Professor, Department of Surgery; Director, Center for Videoendoscopic Surgery, University of Washington, Seattle, Washington

P.A. PARASKEVA, BSc (Hons), MBBS (Hons), PhD, FRCS, Lecturer in Surgery Department of Surgical Oncology and Technology, Imperial College, London, England

CARLOS A. PELLEGRINI, MD, Harry N. Harkins Professor and Chair, Department of Surgery, University of Washington, Seattle, Washington

CHRISTINE J. REN, MD, Assistant Professor, Department of Surgery, New York University School of Medicine, New York, New York

RAUL ROSENTHAL, MD, FACS, Director, The Bariatric Institute; Head, Section of Minimally Invasive Surgery, Department of General and Vascular Surgery, Cleveland Clinic Florida, Weston, Florida

ANTHONY J. SENAGORE, MD, MS, MBA, Krause-Lieberman Chair in Laparoscopic Colorectal Surgery, Department of Colorectal Surgery, Cleveland Clinic Foundation, Cleveland, Ohio

NORIO SHIRAISHI, MD, Department of Surgery I, Faculty of Medicine, Oita University, Oita, Japan

CONRAD H. SIMPFENDORFER, MD, Minimally Invasive Surgery Fellow, Section of Minimally Invasive Surgery, Department of General and Vascular Surgery, Cleveland Clinic Florida, Weston, Florida

SAMUEL SZOMSTEIN, MD, Associate Director, The Bariatric Institute; Section of Minimally Invasive Surgery, Department of General and Vascular Surgery, Cleveland Clinic Florida, Weston, Florida

PATRICIA SYLLA, MD, Postdoctoral Residency Fellow, Department of Surgery, College of Physicians and Surgeons of Columbia University, New York, New York

W.W.C. TSANG, FRCSEd (Gen), Minimal Access Surgery Training Centre, Department of Surgery, Pamela Youde Nethersole Eastern Hospital, Hong Kong

SELMAN URANUES, MD, FACS, Department of Surgery, Medical University of Graz, Graz, Austria

STEVEN D. WEXNER, MD, FACS, FRCS, FRCS (Ed), Chairman, Department of Colorectal Surgery, Cleveland Clinic Florida, Tampa, Florida; Professor of Surgery, Ohio State University Health Sciences Center at the Cleveland Clinic Foundation, Columbus, Ohio; and Clinical Professor of Surgery, University of South Florida College of Medicine, Weston, Florida

RICHARD L. WHELAN, MD, Associate Professor, Department of Surgery, College of Physicians and Surgeons of Columbia University, New York, New York

CONTENTS

Surgical trauma causes significant alterations in host immune function. Compared with open surgery, laparoscopic surgery is associated with reduced postoperative pain and more rapid return to normal activity. Experimental data have also shown more aggressive tumor establishment and growth rates following open surgery than laparoscopic surgery. Surgery-related immunosuppression may be partly responsible for the differences in cancer growth and outcome noted. It is clear that the choice of abdominal surgical approach has immunologic consequences. Further studies are needed to better define the time course and extent of surgery-related alterations in the immune system and their clinical importance. A better understanding of the impact of surgery on the immune system may provide opportunities for pharmacologic manipulation of postoperative immune function to improve clinical results.

Laparoscopic management of sigmoid diverticular disease has emerged as an important adjunct to the armamentarium of surgical options for this disease process. Although there are no prospective randomized studies directly comparing laparoscopic and open colectomy for diverticulitis, the comparative studies provide compelling data. The magnitude of the benefits achieved with laparoscopic colectomy in the hands of experienced laparoscopic colon surgeons may soon be sufficient to make laparoscopic colectomy the standard of care.

to examine long-term efficacy, with a high priority given to randomized controlled trials.

Since 1991, laparoscopic surgery has been adopted for the treatment of gastric tumors, including gastric cancer and gastric gastrointestinal submucosal tumor (GIST). Although laparoscopic gastric resection for gastric tumors has not been accepted worldwide, its use has definitively increased due to its reduced invasiveness. The most common procedures are laparoscopy-assisted distal gastrectomy (LADG) for cancer and laparoscopic local resection for GIST. To establish laparoscopic gastric resection as a standard of care for gastric tumors, multicenter randomized controlled clinical trials are needed to evaluate its short- and long-term outcomes.

FORTHCOMING ISSUES

RECENT ISSUES

The Clinics are now available online!

www.theclinics.com

ELSEVIER
SAUNDERS

SURGICAL
CLINICS OF
NORTH AMERICA

Surg Clin N Am 85 (2005) xiii–xiv

Preface

Laparoscopic Surgery: Beyond Mere Feasibility

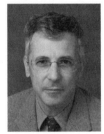

Nilesh A. Patel, MD   Roberto Bergamaschi, MD, PhD
Guest Editors

An increasing number of surgeons are routinely performing advanced laparoscopic surgery, as witnessed by the literature published since the early 1990s. Some papers are case series without controls and are thus capable only of suggesting feasibility. Comparison papers claim the superiority of laparoscopic surgery against conventional surgery based on improvements in postoperative ileus, timing of food resumption, or length of hospital stay. However, these are surrogate end points, because they are not a direct measure of the clinical outcome of the surgical procedure. For example, length of stay may depend more on preoperative counseling, discharge criteria, social arrangements, patients' health literacy, or type of health system than the means of surgical access. The question of whether laparoscopic surgery should be considered the standard of care can only be answered by measuring clinical outcome measures, which are a direct measure of either harm or clinical benefit. Examples of clinical outcome measures include decreased rates of small bowel obstruction, incisional hernia, or disease-specific recurrence as well as improvements in abdominal wall scarring.

An attempt has been made in this issue of the *Surgical Clinics of North America* to provide readers with concise insight into the evidence available in support of routinely performed advanced laparoscopic procedures such as bariatric operations, colorectal or gastric resections, surgery of the spleen, and paraesophageal and ventral hernia repair. This issue is not meant to

doi:10.1016/j.suc.2004.11.001   surgical.theclinics.com

offer a comprehensive review of nonadvanced procedures (eg, cholecystectomy, repair of inguinal hernia, fundoplication, and so forth) or of nonroutine advanced procedures (eg, donor nephrectomy, pancreatic tail resection, and so forth). Rather, it highlights relevant immunologic advantages and addresses what clinical benefit or harm can be expected from routinely performed advanced laparoscopic procedures.

We hope that readers enjoy this issue, take the challenge to heart, and strive to answer the questions it raises. We would like to thank all of the authors for generously contributing their time and expertise. We would also like to acknowledge Catherine Bewick of Elsevier for her tremendous support and assistance in bringing this issue to fruition in addition to the honor of serving as Guest Editors for the *Surgical Clinics of North America.*

Nilesh A. Patel, MD
Divisions of Bariatric and General Surgery
Department of Surgery
Allegheny General Hospital
320 East North Avenue
Pittsburgh, PA 15212, USA

E-mail address: npatel@wpahs.org

Roberto Bergamaschi, MD, PhD, FRCS, FASCRS, FACS
Minimally Invasive Surgery Center and Program
Allegheny General Hospital
320 East North Avenue
Pittsburgh, PA 15212, USA

E-mail address: rbergama@wpahs.org

ELSEVIER
SAUNDERS

SURGICAL
CLINICS OF
NORTH AMERICA

Surg Clin N Am 85 (2005) 1–18

Immunological advantages of advanced laparoscopy

Patricia Sylla, MD, Irena Kirman, MD, PhD,
Richard L. Whelan, MD*

*Department of Surgery, College of Physicians and Surgeons of Columbia University,
630 West 168th Street, New York, NY 10032, USA*

Traditional major open abdominal operations have potent effects on the immune system. Specifically, surgical trauma induces an inflammatory state characterized by the release of pro-inflammatory cytokines and acute-phase proteins. Surgical manipulation also depresses cell-mediated immunity manifested by alterations in the recruitment, activation, and function of circulating lymphocytes, monocytes, and other immune cells. The extent of these effects is proportional to the magnitude of the surgical procedure. During the last 15 years, advanced laparoscopic techniques have revolutionized general surgery. Relative to conventional open surgery, minimally invasive surgery is associated with reduced postoperative pain, more prompt return of bowel function, reduced hospital stay, and more rapid return to normal activity, as reflected by multiple prospective randomized clinical trials [1–7]. These short-term clinical benefits are generally attributed to the lesser degree of abdominal wall trauma incurred by laparoscopic procedures. Does significantly limiting injury to the abdominal wall influence the immune response? Stated differently, does the choice of abdominal access (laparotomy versus pneumoperitoneum/laparoscopy) impact postoperative immune function, despite the fact that what is done inside the abdomen is the same? To answer these questions, a significant body of research has developed since the advent of minimally invasive surgery.

Some might question the relevance of postoperative immunosuppression. Admittedly, there are few data regarding the clinical ramifications of postoperative immunosuppression after major operations in immunocompetent individuals. There is information regarding surgical morbidity in

---

* Corresponding author.
E-mail address: rlw3@columbia.edu (R.L. Whelan).

doi:10.1016/j.suc.2004.09.005

patients who are significantly immunosuppressed before surgery, however. Anergic patients and those on immunosuppressive medications have a higher rate of postoperative infections and other morbidities than immunocompetent patients [8]. Thus, one can infer that the temporary immunosuppression attendant to major abdominal surgery may increase the chances of postoperative infection. It is also important to note that anergic cancer patients undergoing attempted curative resection of their primary tumors are more likely to have unresectable tumors, as well as a higher recurrence rate and mortality, than immunocompetent patients who have similar tumors. Finally, colectomy patients who received perioperative transfusions, a known cause of cell-mediated immunosuppression, have a worse long-term outcome than nontransfused patients who has the same disease stage [9]. The fact that immunosuppressed patients have a poorer oncologic outcome after surgery suggests that surgery-related immunosuppression might significantly impact a patient's innate defenses against the formation of metastases.

In addition to the above literature regarding immune function after open and closed surgery, there is also a body of work, both human and experimental, regarding tumor growth after surgery. Although factors besides immunosuppression may influence tumor cell survival and establishment of metastases, these studies merit our attention, especially in light of the conflicting cancer outcome results from two randomized colectomy trials. Lacy et al [6] reported a significant survival benefit for the laparoscopic-assisted group, with a median follow up of 43 months. The 2004 National Cancer Institute (NCI)-sponsored Clinical Outcomes of Surgical Therapy (COST) study, with a median follow up of 4.4 years, however, reported no significant differences in survival or recurrence between the open and closed colectomy groups [7]. Thus, despite concern and controversy regarding port-site tumors and the appropriateness of minimally invasive methods in the setting of cancer, results suggest that laparoscopic methods are associated with either similar or possibly better cancer outcome. The oncologic basic science literature in this area may shed some light on this subject.

This article reviews the literature in this evolving field. As will become evident, although there are measurable differences in immune parameters between the two surgical methods, the clinical significance of these short-term differences have not been clearly established. Likewise, although there are animal and limited human data suggesting that minimally invasive methods are associated with a postoperative state conducive to increased tumor growth, at this time there are limited long-term data supporting this position.

Systemic inflammatory response

Like other conditions associated with tissue injury, such as infection, burns, and trauma, surgery evokes a potent local and systemic inflammatory response manifested by rapid changes in the plasma concentration of various acute-phase proteins and pro-inflammatory cytokines. Although increased levels of cytokines and acute-phase proteins reflect an inflammatory response, they do not directly correlate with the status of the immune system. The literature in this area demonstrates that in both burn injury associated with sepsis and in blunt trauma, serum concentrations of IL-6, IL-8, and TNFα are increased, and these elevations are associated with an increased risk of infectious complications [10] and overall morbidity [10–12]. Consequently, excessive activation secondary to these inflammatory mediators [13] has been viewed by some investigators and clinicians as indicative of a state of tolerance to specific immune stimuli.

Plasma levels of acute phase proteins such as C-reactive protein (CRP), the most widely measured marker of the acute-phase response, and the pro-inflammatory cytokines IL-1β, IL-6, IL-8, and TNFα are typically transiently increased following significant tissue injury. IL-6 has been consistently found to be transiently increased in response to injury. Pre- and postoperative plasma levels of the above inflammatory mediators have been compared in patients undergoing laparoscopic and conventional surgery. Reports on the stress response following open and laparoscopic surgery have shown that open cholecystectomy is associated with higher postoperative plasma levels of CRP, TNFα, IL-1β, and IL-6 relative to laparoscopic cholecystectomy, suggesting that open surgery is associated with a greater inflammatory response [14–20]. Significantly higher levels of some or all of these proteins were also found postoperatively following conventional Nissen fundoplication [21,22] and colorectal cancer resection relative to the equivalent laparoscopic operations [23–25]. Other studies have shown that although both open and laparoscopic colorectal surgery are associated with elevated plasma CRP levels, there is more prompt return to baseline preoperative values following the latter [26]. Many of these studies, however, indicate that postoperative differences in the levels of these inflammatory cytokines between open and laparoscopic procedures are short-lived, with differences most pronounced 1 to 6 hours postoperatively and no longer detectable by postoperative day 2 [20,24,25]. Furthermore, other studies have failed to find any difference in postoperative levels of these markers after laparoscopic and open colorectal cancer resection [27–29], or between laparoscopic and open cholecystectomy performed via a minilaparotomy [30]. These variable results have been attributed by some to the small size and nonrandomized nature of the above studies, the timing of postoperative blood sampling, and the fact that some populations studied contained both cancer patients and patients who have benign disorders. Several prospective randomized studies comparing postoperative changes in levels of acute-phase proteins following laparoscopic cholecystectomy [31], herniorrhaphy [32], or laparoscopic-assisted colorectal resection for non-cancerous lesions [33] with their open counterparts showed no significant differences between groups. These inconsistent findings may be due to the variable degree of tissue trauma incurred by specific types of surgery. Of note, the majority of cholecsytectomy studies comparing inflammatory marker levels found lower levels following the laparoscopic approach [14–20]. Most of the conflicting results are found in herniorrhaphy or colectomy studies that compared open and closed methods.

In regards to herniorrhaphy, it is not surprising that few, if any, perturbations are noted, because neither the open nor closed operations incur much tissue damage. Laparoscopic-assisted colorectal resections, on the other hand, require an incision substantially larger than that typically required for other advanced laparoscopic procedures, such as gastric bypass or anti-reflux procedures. Some have suggested that the differences in cytokine response noted after laparoscopic operations are related to the extent of abdominal wall trauma, and thus one would anticipate less marked differences following laparoscopic-assisted colectomy. Further, in regards to colectomy, there is a wide variation in the size of the incision needed to extract the specimen and facilitate the anastamosis, dependent on body habitus, the size of the specimen, and the surgeon. Unfortunately, a substantial proportion of colectomy studies do not provide detailed information regarding incision length. In addition, there is no consensus amongst surgeons as to what constitutes a laparoscopic-assisted procedure or conversion. Other variables that may impact the results of cytokine studies include blood transfusions and the extent and location (right versus left) of the bowel resection performed. Therefore, when evaluating the systemic inflammatory response, the colectomy population is much more heterogeneous in regards to procedure performed and abdominal wall trauma induced than other advanced procedures.

To summarize, with some notable exceptions, the majority of studies suggest that the systemic stress response, as judged by the levels of cytokines and acute phase proteins, is significantly less robust after minimally invasive procedures. These are mostly short-lived differences. It is critical to note that the clinical implications of these differences, where they exist, have not been determined. To assess immune function after surgery, it is more logical to study the cell-mediated immune response, which involves the coordinated activation of critical subsets of immune cells in response to specific local and systemic challenges.

Cell-mediated immunity

Cell-mediated immunity is involved in clearing infectious agents and in tumor defense. Tissue injury, including surgical trauma, inhibits the cellular immune response [34]. In addition to altering serum cytokine levels, surgery induces changes in the numbers and subsets of circulating immune cells, and may alter proliferation rates and activation of lymphocytes and other immune cells [35]. Specifically, some have noted that surgical manipulation is associated with increased postoperative leukocyte and neutrophil counts [36] and decreased peripheral lymphocyte counts [34,37], both proportional in magnitude to the degree of surgical trauma [36]. Postoperatively, alterations in the proportion or function of macrophages and monocytes, as well as lymphocyte subsets such as T cells and natural killer (NK) cells, have been described [35,37,38]. CD4 helper T lymphocytes are decreased in number relative to cytotoxic CD8 cells. Th1 helper cells, which activate the cellular immune response, are proportionally reduced relative to Th2 cells, favoring the humoral response through B-cell stimulation. This decline in the CD4/CD8 and Th1/Th2 ratios has been well documented following surgical stress [37,39]. In addition, in a clinical study by Hensler and colleagues [40], both T-cell proliferation and IL-2, IL-4, INFγ, and TNFα cytokine production in response to T-cell receptor activation via CD3/CD28 crosslinking were transiently inhibited in the early postoperative period following major open surgery, suggesting T-cell hyporesponsiveness to mitogenic stimuli.

Clinical studies comparing the effects of open and laparoscopic surgery on the various components of cell-mediated immunity have shown more significant alterations in peripheral leukocyte counts in patients following open surgery, with higher counts following open cholecystectomy [31,36,41] and open colorectal resection [24] relative to patients undergoing equivalent laparoscopic procedures. In patients undergoing laparoscopic procedures, there is also a more rapid return to preoperative leukocyte counts than in open surgery patients [25]. Other studies, however, describe no significant differences in leukocyte numbers following open cholecystectomy [26], open Nissen fundoplication [21], or open colorectal resection [29] relative to the respective laparoscopic groups.

When lymphocyte counts were evaluated, open cholecystectomy and colectomy were associated with more profound and prolonged decreases in total lymphocyte numbers than laparoscopic counterparts [16,26,42,43]. Examination of the changes in relative proportions of lymphocyte subsets in response to surgery has also revealed significant differences between open and minimally invasive procedures. Higher postoperative CD4/CD8 ratios attributed to relatively preserved CD4 helper T-cell counts were described following laparoscopic colorectal surgery [26,43]. In contrast to open surgery patients who showed postoperative inhibition of Th1 function—evidenced by reduced production of IL-2, INFγ, and TNFα—patients undergoing laparoscopic cholecystectomy [39,42,44] and laparoscopic gastrectomy [45] demonstrated preserved Th1 function and more vigorous Th2 activity.

Other lymphocyte subsets such as CD31+ T cells and NK cells, which play an important role in T-cell migration to the periphery, are differentially affected by surgical modalities. In a clinical study, NK cell counts were reduced following open but not laparoscopic cholecystectomy [42,43]. CD31 plays an important role in lymphocyte-endothelial adhesion. Comparison of the proportion of pre- and postoperative circulating CD31+ T cells in patients undergoing either laparoscopic or open colorectal surgery showed a significantly smaller proportion of CD31+ T cells in the open group on postoperative days 1 and 3 [46]. This relative decrease in CD31+ T cells correlated with the length of incision, suggesting impaired T-cell migration from the circulation to the periphery following open surgery [46]. Several studies examining the differential effects of laparoscopic and open colorectal surgery on circulating lymphocytes, however, found no significant differences in lymphocyte counts and CD4 to CD8 ratios [24,25,27–29,47]. It is unclear whether these conflicting findings are related to the type of surgery under investigation or to other factors.

In-vitro lymphocyte proliferation in response to mitogens or superantigens was better preserved following laparoscopic than open cholecystectomy [48,49]. One animal study compared the effects of laparotomy and CO_2 pneumoperitoneum on splenic T-lymphocyte proliferation in response to mitogen stimulation. Relative to anesthesia, proliferation of splenic T lymphocytes on postoperative days (POD) 2 to 4 was preserved following pneumoperitoneum but reduced following laparotomy [50].

NK cells are an important lymphocyte subset involved in cellular and tumor immunity, and postoperative NK cell cytotoxicity was markedly suppressed in cancer patients following open surgical resection [51]. In an animal study [52], postoperative inhibition of NK cell activity following laparotomy correlated with increased growth of implanted tumors. In a different study [45,53], NK cell cytotoxicity and lymphocyte-activated killer cell (LAK) activity (highly potent tumoricidal cells generated by IL-1β- and IFNγ-induced stimulation of NK cells) were more profoundly suppressed in mice following laparotomy than CO_2 pneumoperitoneum [53]. Only two clinical studies to date have specifically compared the effects of laparoscopic versus open surgery on NK cell activity. There were no significant differences noted when NK cell cytotoxicity was compared after open and laparoscopic cholecystectomy; similarly, no differences were found following laparoscopic and open colorectal resection [54].

Because of their central role in both innate and cell-mediated immunity, the differential effects of laparoscopic and open surgery on monocyte and macrophage activities have been extensively evaluated in clinical studies. When comparing macrophage and monocyte phagocytic and enzymatic function between laparoscopic and conventional surgery, postoperative chemotaxis and production of TNFα and superoxide anion were significantly decreased following open cholecystectomy, but preserved following laparoscopic cholecystectomy [31]. Upon in-vitro stimulation with lipopolysaccharide (LPS), postoperative mononuclear cell production of IL-6 and TNFα was reduced in patients undergoing open colorectal resection and preserved in laparoscopic patients [24]. Macrophages and Polymorphonuclear cells (PMNs) from patients undergoing open cholecystectomy showed a significant reduction in phagocytosis and killing of *Candida albicans* in vitro relative to the results observed in patients undergoing laparoscopic cholecystectomy [55]. Another study, however, found no significant differences in the same parameters between patients undergoing either open or laparoscopic cholecystectomy [56].

Due to their ability to recognize, process, and present foreign antigens, mononuclear cells also play a central role in cell-mediated immunity. The magnitude of monocyte downregulation of HLA-DR expression in patients following major surgical trauma correlated with an increased risk of postoperative sepsis, likely due to impaired antigen-presenting function [57–59]. The effect of laparoscopic versus open surgery on monocyte HLA-DR expression has been compared in several clinical studies. Several non-randomized studies found significantly decreased expression at a variety of times ranging from POD 1 to 8 following open surgery. No alterations were found in monocytes from patients undergoing laparoscopic surgery [15,47]. Other prospective randomized studies comparing monocyte HLA-DR expression in patients undergoing open and closed cholecystectomy, Nissen fundoplication or colorectal resection found decreased HLA-DR expression in both operative groups after surgery; however, more profound and long-lasting changes were noted in the open groups for each of these procedures [21,24,43,44]. Of note, several other clinical studies reported no differences between laparoscopic and open colorectal procedures in the degree or extent of depression of HLA-DR expression on mononuclear cells [25,29,33].

Although there are conflicting results for numerous parameters, overall, in the opinion of the authors, the data suggest that open surgery is associated with a greater degree of immune imbalance than laparoscopic surgery. The reasons for the inconsistencies noted between the clinical studies are unclear. There is a great degree of variation in the patient populations evaluated, postoperative sampling time points, and assays used to assess the same parameters across studies. In the case of colectomy, variations in the size of the incision used for specimen removal as well as whether the abdominal muscles are split or divided in making the incision may account for some of the differences noted. It should also be noted that differences in cell numbers and surface antigen expression do not necessarily reflect alterations in their function. Serial delayed type hypersensitivity (DTH) testing perioperatively provides an assessment of cell-mediated immune function that perhaps provides more meaningful data.

Delayed-type hypersensitivity response and T cell-specific function

DTH testing to recall antigens provides an indirect assessment of multiple elements of the immune system, all of which must be functioning for a positive response to be generated. The afferent arm of the response requires that an antigen-presenting cell process and present the antigen to a CD4+ memory T cell. The efferent arm involves proliferation of the stimulated CD4+ T-cell and cytokine elaboration. Finally, immune effector cells must gather at the site of challenge, after which fibrin is deposited and edema and induration develop. Comparison of DTH response size to the same recall antigen, injected both pre- and postoperatively, provides a means of assessing the functional status of the immune system. Major open surgery results in a significant but temporary decrease in the size of the DTH response, which is thought to be a manifestation of partial suppression of the immune system [34,60]. This effect has been reported to persist for 6 to 9 days after major open abdominal procedures [60,61].

Although this temporary decrease or loss of DTH response after surgery has not been associated with a higher rate of complications, there are data regarding anergic patients who cannot mount a DTH response pre- or postoperatively. As mentioned above, in surgical patients who have [62] or do not have malignancies [63,64], preoperative anergy has been associated with increased rates of postoperative sepsis and mortality and increased tumor recurrence [65]. Pre- and postoperative DTH response to skin antigens has been compared following open versus laparoscopic surgery in animal and clinical studies. Animal studies have found CO_2 pneumoperitoneum to be associated with significantly better preservation of the DTH response than open surgery [66–70]. In addition, in a study evaluating cellular immunity by measuring both DTH response and rejection of implanted immunogenic tumors in mice, animals undergoing laparotomy showed a significantly impaired DTH response and ability to reject tumors postoperatively relative to mice subjected to CO_2 pneumoperitoneum, in which both parameters were better preserved [71]. A human cholecystectomy study that included a POD 1 and POD 6 DTH challenge noted a significant reduction in DTH response on POD 1, but not at the latter time point in the open patients. In contrast, the laparoscopic patients' postoperative responses were not significantly different from preoperative results [15]. In a study comparing open and minimally invasive colorectal resection, DTH challenges were given immediately following the operation and on POD 3. Significantly smaller responses were noted at both time points in the open patients, whereas no such differences were found in the laparoscopic group [72]. Neither study correlated the DTH responses with clinical end points.

Clinical data have shown that, in contrast to laparoscopic surgery, open surgery reduces HLA-DR expression on mononuclear cells relative to preoperative levels. These data suggest a possible mechanism for cell-mediated immunosuppression following surgical trauma, whereby open surgery, by reducing HLA-DR expression on monocytes, impairs antigen presentation with subsequently reduced T-cell activation. Two clinical studies to date [40,44], however, have shown that although circulating monocytes from patients undergoing open cholecystectomy have significantly reduced expression of HLA-DR antigens postoperatively, activation of T cells by bacterial superantigens was preserved. The authors of the studies concluded that loss of HLA-DR may not affect antigen-presenting capacity of antigen presenting cells (APCs), or that loading of very few MHC II molecules with superantigens may be sufficient to stimulate T-cell proliferation [40,44].

Data on the effect of surgery on T cells (open and laparoscopic) have focused on postoperative T-cell counts, changes in proportion of different lymphocyte subsets, and lymphocyte proliferation in response to mitogens. Only one study has evaluated, in a more specific manner, the effect of major open surgery on T-cell proliferation. The proliferative response of T cells isolated from postoperative plasma was evaluated after CD3 ligation and CD28 receptors, and was found to be transiently but significantly reduced relative to preoperative plasma samples [40]. Therefore, defective signaling through the T-cell receptor/CD3 and CD28 complex may represent an important mechanism of immunosuppression following surgery.

Some insight into the specific molecular effects of laparotomy and laparoscopy on T cells comes from a microarray analysis on the time course of the differential effects of sham laparotomy versus CO_2 pneumo-peritoneum on splenic T-cell gene expression in mice (Sylla et al, submitted for publication, 2004). Relative to anesthesia control, 12 hours after surgery, sham laparotomy resulted in notable alterations in 398 T-cell genes compared with 116 genes following pneumoperitoneum. At 24 hours the differences between the two surgical methods were less marked, with alterations in expression noted in 157 genes following laparotomy, as opposed to 132 genes after pneumoperitoneum. When global gene expression was compared between laparotomy and pneumoperitoneum, expression of 177 genes was increased following laparotomy relative to pneumoperitoneum at 12 hours, a difference that was reduced fourfold at the 24-hour time point (Sylla et al, submitted for publication, 2004). Functional differences in gene expression between 12 and 24 hours after surgery were also noted in both groups. These transient but substantial alterations in splenic T-cell gene expression profiles following laparotomy provide a molecular basis for the observation that open surgery is associated with transient but marked immune alterations. Ongoing functional analysis of those genes with differential expression in response to laparotomy and pneumoperitoneum will not only uncover the biological significance of these differences, but may identify genes that can be used as clinical markers of the effect of surgery on the immune system (Sylla et al, submitted for publication, 2004).

Overall, data from both animal and clinical studies have shown better preservation of cell-mediated immunity response following laparoscopic relative to open surgery, as reflected by preserved DTH response and T-cell proliferation. Although both procedures have a potent effect on splenic T-cell gene expression, pneumoperitoneum is associated with fewer alterations in gene expression than laparotomy. No clinical study has yet determined the clinical consequences of diminished DTH responses or the alterations mentioned above. These differences have not been linked to differences in postoperative infections or other complications, and thus their clinical significance is not presently clear. Additional studies are needed to determine the effect of the various immune system perturbations that have been noted on clinical outcomes.

Peritoneal macrophage function

Because of their role in the local cellular response and systemic inflammatory response to abdominal trauma, the effect of surgery and pneumoperitoneum on peritoneal macrophages has been investigated, largely in animal studies. Macrophages play an important role in cellular immunity. Through expression of major histocompatibility complex antigens (MHC), macrophages mediate activation and amplification of T cell-specific responses. In addition to their tumoricidal activity, demonstrated in vitro and in vivo [73], macrophages also function in phagocytosis, production of cytotoxic molecules, and tumor cell lysis. The following parameters have been used as markers of macrophage activation: expression of MHC Class II antigen and production of superoxide anion, hydrogen peroxide, nitric oxide, TNFα, and IL-6 [55]. In mice undergoing laparotomy, Redmond and coauthors [74] described postoperative impairment of peritoneal macrophage antigen-presenting function and microbicidal activity, as manifested by impaired surface Ia expression, reduced phagocytosis and killing of Candida albicans, and reduced superoxide release in response to phorbol myristate acetate (PMA), with return to baseline function on POD 3.

Peritoneal macrophage studies have compared open and closed surgical methods, reporting conflicting results. One animal study found laparoscopic, but not open, Nissen fundoplication to be associated with enhanced bacterial clearance by peritoneal macrophages [75], and another found production of hydrogen peroxide in response to PMA to be reduced following open but not laparoscopic cecectomy [76]. The results of all other studies to date have conflicted with these findings. Specifically, production of TNFα and IL-1β [77], nitric oxide (NO), and inducible NO synthase (iNOS) by peritoneal macrophages [78] in response to lipopolysaccharide (LPS) stimulation were impaired following laparoscopy, but preserved following either gasless laparoscopy or laparotomy. In addition, CO_2 pneumoperitoneum was associated with postoperative impairment of bacterial clearance [79,80], cytokine production [81,82], phagocytic activity, and cytotoxic activity against tumor cells [83] relative to either helium, air insufflation, or laparotomy. In-vitro studies on the specific effects of CO_2 on macrophages found that in addition to reducing intra-abdominal pH to a greater extent than air or helium [84], CO_2 pneumoperitoneum results in the cytosolic acidification of peritoneal macrophages, which correlates with decreased LPS-induced TNFα production [85]. Given these conflicting findings, further investigation of the role of peritoneal macrophages in the local immune response to surgery and cancer and studies on the molecular mechanisms involved in peritoneal macrophage impairment by CO_2 are necessary.

Immune surveillance in tumor resistance and the effect of surgical stress

The role of the immune system in natural tumor resistance has been long debated. Clinical and experimental evidence supports the concept that the immune system, especially T cells, plays a role in antitumor defense. Immunocompromised patients are at higher risk of tumor development, and immunodeficient animals exhibit higher rate of spontaneous and induced tumors than wild-type controls. Using experimental models of breast and colon cancer, tumors have been shown to inhibit maturation of T- and B-cell precursors, or to deplete newly developing lymphocytes [86–90]. Immune function can be further compromised by the impact of surgical trauma. Surgery-induced inflammation induces activation of inflammatory cells such as granulocytes, monocytes, and lymphocytes. Nonspecific activation is known to be followed by apoptosis, which has been demonstrated for mononuclear cells and granulocytes. Surgery-related inflammatory response may further deplete immune resources and aggravate tumor-related immune alterations. Thus, surgical trauma modifies major components of host defense and affects tumor resistance mechanisms. Consequences of surgery-related inflammation most certainly affect the development of antigen-specific cells and alter the balance of cell-growth regulatory and angiogenesis-stimulatory factors, and may result in the inhibition of tumor resistance. It is hoped that future studies will identify specific targets implicated in the reaction to surgical stress, leading to new treatment strategies that will improve the outcome of surgery.

The impact of surgery on tumor resistance

The effects of open and laparoscopic surgery on tumor resistance have been compared in experimental models. Numerous experimental studies have demonstrated that laparotomy, when compared with CO_2 pneumo-peritoneum or anesthesia alone, is associated with increased tumor establishment and growth [91–94]. Similar results were noted after open and closed bowel resection [95]. Tumor-cell proliferation was increased and apoptosis decreased after laparotomy in a murine study [96]. The mechanism of these growth differences has also been investigated. Laparotomy-related inhibition of cell-mediated immune function may account for some of the observed differences in tumor growth after surgery in the experimental setting [52,97].

Both open and laparoscopic procedures involve traumatic handling of tumor tissue, with a subsequent release of liberated tumor cells. Furthermore, surgical trauma shifts the balance of growth-stimulatory/

growth-inhibitory soluble factors, which may support the growth and establishment of liberated tumor cells. Finally, the process of operative intervention induces a powerful inflammatory reaction that engages immune cells in nonspecific activation and subsequent apoptosis. Thus, tumor recurrence following surgery may be linked to the above-mentioned factors, namely, a surge of liberated tumor cells, altered balance of growth-stimulatory/growth-inhibitory soluble substances, and altered immune function.

Modulation of tumor growth-stimulatory/growth-regulatory factors following surgery

Surgical trauma has been shown to induce activation of proteases, which subsequently degrade cell-growth regulatory factors susceptible to proteolysis, such as insulinlike growth-factor binding protein 3 (IGFBP-3) [98,99]. IGFBP-3 is known to inhibit the growth of breast, lung, prostate, and colon cancer cells [100–103]. The growth of transformed colonic epithelial cells is suppressed by IGFBP-3 in vitro and in experimental models [103,104]. Although the intact IGFBP-3 molecule induces apoptosis of many types of tumor cells, its degradation products lack this activity [105]. Surgery-associated inflammatory processes are likely to activate IGFBP-3 proteolysis. The authors have demonstrated that the extent of IGFBP-3 depletion following open surgery correlates with an increased concentration of the pro-inflammatory cytokine IL-6 [106], which might merely be a correlative marker or inducer of IGFBP-3 proteolysis. We have also shown that open but not laparoscopic surgery induces a significant decrease in the level of intact IGFBP-3. In general, approximately 80% of open colectomies and 30% of laparoscopic procedures are followed by substantial IGFBP-3 depletion [107]. Further, we demonstrated that POD 1 serum from open surgery patients stimulated in-vitro tumor growth when compared with the same patients' preoperative blood samples. Of note, POD 1 blood from laparoscopic patients did not stimulate in-vitro tumor growth beyond that observed in cultures into which preoperative serum from these same patients had been added. Future clinical trials will determine whether there is an association between postoperative IGFBP-3 depletion and colon cancer recurrence. Currently, we can conclude that open and not minimally invasive surgery leads to a significant depletion of the important cell-growth regulatory protein IGFBP-3.

Summary

Surgical trauma clearly results in deleterious alterations in immune function. The bulk of the available data suggests that minimally invasive methods, when compared with results following open procedures, are associated with significantly less pronounced perturbations in immune function. This is true for a number of pro-inflammatory cytokines, acute-phase proteins, DTH response, and at least one growth-regulatory factor. There are conflicting data, however, concerning many of these parameters, and it is critical to note that the documented postoperative alterations have not been definitely associated with specific complications or differences in clinical outcomes. It is possible that improved overall immune function following laparoscopic surgery accounts for some of the short-term clinical benefits that have been well documented. Laparotomy clearly impacts postoperative tumor growth in the experimental setting. This may or may not be related to surgery-related changes in immune function. There are clinical data demonstrating alterations in levels and activity of some serum growth factors following surgery that may also impact on postoperative tumor growth. Overall, evaluation of perioperative immune function warrants further investigation. Further studies should provide us with a better understanding of the impact of surgery on the host, and hold the promise of new therapeutic targets and pharmacologic methods to manipulate the host immune response perioperatively so as to minimize complications, and perhaps improve long-term oncologic results in the setting of cancer.

References

[1] Memon MA, Cooper NJ, Memon B, et al. Meta-analysis of randomized clinical trials comparing open and laparoscopic inguinal hernia repair. Br J Surg 2003;90(12):1479–92.

[2] Ortega AE, Hunter JG, Peters JH, et al. A prospective, randomized comparison of laparoscopic appendectomy with open appendectomy. Laparoscopic appendectomy study group. Am J Surg 1995;169(2):208–12.

[3] McMahon AJ, Russell IT, Baxter JN, et al. Laparoscopic versus minilaparotomy cholecystectomy: a randomized trial. Lancet 1994;343(8890):135–8.

[4] Milsom JW, Hammerhofer KA, Bohm B, et al. Prospective, randomized trial comparing laparoscopic vs. conventional surgery for refractory ileocolic Crohn's disease. Dis Colon Rectum 2001;44(1):1–8.

[5] Milsom JW, Bohm B, Hammerhofer KA, et al. A prospective, randomized trial comparing laparoscopic versus conventional techniques in colorectal cancer surgery: a preliminary report. J Am Coll Surg 1998;187(1):46–54.

[6] Lacy AM, Garcia-Valdecasas JC, Delgado S, et al. Laparoscopy-assisted colectomy versus open colectomy for treatment of non-metastatic colon cancer: a randomized trial. Lancet 2002;359(9325):2224–9.

[7] Clinical Outcomes of Surgical Therapy Study Group. A comparison of laparoscopically assisted and open colectomy for colon cancer. N Engl J Med 2004;350(20):2050–9.

[8] Liu AY, Wagner WO, Piedmonte MR, et al. Anergic response to delayed hypersensitivity skin testing. A predictor of early mortality in heart transplant recipients. Chest 1993;104(6):1668–72.

[9] Foster RS, Costanza MC, Foster JC, et al. Adverse relationship between blood transfusions and survival after colectomy for colon cancer. Cancer 1985;55(6):1195–201.

[10] Drost AC, Burleson DG, Cioffi WG, et al. Plasma cytokines after thermal injury and their relationship to infection. Ann Surg 1993;218(1):74–8.

[11] Yamada Y, Endo S, Inada K. Plasma cytokine levels in patients with severe burn injury—with reference to the relationship between infection and prognosis. Burns 1996; 22(8):587–93.

[12] Roumen RM, Hendriks T, van der Ven-Jongekrijg J, et al. Cytokine patterns in patients after major vascular surgery, hemorrhagic shock, and severe blunt trauma. Relation with subsequent adult respiratory distress syndrome and multiple organ failure. Ann Surg 1993; 218(6):769–76.

[13] Epstein FH. Acute-phase proteins and other systemic responses to inflammation. N Engl J Med 1999;340(6):448–54.

[14] Jakeways MS, Mitchell V, Hashim IA, et al. Metabolic and inflammatory responses after open or laparoscopic cholecystectomy. Br J Surg 1994;81(1):127–31.

[15] Kloosterman T, von Blomberg BM, Borgstein P, et al. Unimpaired immune functions after laparoscopic cholecystectomy. Surgery 1994;115(4):424–8.

[16] Dionigi R, Dominioni L, Benevento A, et al. Effects of surgical trauma of laparoscopic vs. open cholecystectomy. Hepatogastroenterology 1994;41(5):471–6.

[17] Karayiannakis AJ, Makri GG, Mantzioka A, et al. Systemic stress response after laparoscopic or open cholecystectomy: a randomized trial. Br J Surg 1997;84(4):467–71.

[18] Bruce DM, Smith M, Walker CB, et al. Minimal access surgery for cholelithiasis induces an attenuated acute phase response. Am J Surg 1999;178(3):232–4.

[19] Squirrell DM, Majeed AW, Troy G, et al. A randomized, prospective, blinded comparison of postoperative pain, metabolic response, and perceived health after laparoscopic and small incision cholecystectomy. Surgery 1998;123(5):485–95.

[20] Schietroma M, Carlei F, Mownah A, et al. Changes in the blood coagulation, fibrinolysis, and cytokine profile during laparoscopic and open cholecystectomy. Surg Endosc 2004; 18(7):1090–6.

[21] Sietses C, Wiezer MJ, Eijsbouts QA, et al. A prospective randomized study of the systemic immune response after laparoscopic and conventional Nissen fundoplication. Surgery 1999;126(1):5–9.

[22] Perttila J, Salo M, Ovaska J, et al. Immune response after laparoscopic and conventional Nissen fundoplication. Eur J Surg 1999;165(1):21–8.

[23] Leung KL, Lai PB, Ho RL, et al. Systemic cytokine response after laparoscopic-assisted resection of rectosigmoid carcinoma: a prospective randomized trial. Ann Surg 2000; 231(4):506–11.

[24] Ordemann J, Jacobi CA, Schwenk W, et al. Cellular and humoral inflammatory response after laparoscopic and conventional colorectal resections. Surg Endosc 2001; 15(6):600–8.

[25] Wu FP, Sietses C, von Blomberg BME, et al. Systemic and peritoneal inflammatory response after laparoscopic or conventional colon resection in cancer patients. Dis Colon Rectum 2003;46(2):147–55.

[26] Braga M, Vignali A, Zuliani W, et al. Metabolic and functional results after laparoscopic colorectal surgery. Dis Colon Rectum 2002;45(8):1070–7.

[27] Mehigan BJ, Hartley JE, Drew PJ, et al. Changes in T cell subsets, interleukin-6, and C-reactive protein after laparoscopic and open colorectal resection for malignancy. Surg Endosc 2001;15(11):1289–93.

[28] Tang CL, Eu KW, Tai BC, et al. Randomized clinical trial of the effect of open versus laparoscopically assisted colectomy on systemic immunity in patients with colorectal cancer. Br J Surg 2001;88(6):801–7.

[29] Hewitt PM, Ip SM, Kwok SP, et al. Laproscopic-assisted vs. open surgery for colorectal cancer, comparative study of immune effects. Dis Colon Rectum 1998;41(7):901–9.

[30] McMahon AJ, O'Dwyer PJ, Cruikshank AM, et al. Comparison of metabolic responses to laparoscopic and minilaparotomy cholecystectomy. Br J Surg 1993;80(10):1255–8.

[31] Redmond HP, Watson RW, Houghton T, et al. Immune function in patients undergoing open vs laparoscopic cholecystectomy. Arch Surg 1994;129(12):1240–6.

[32] Hill AD, Banwell PE, Darzi A, et al. Inflammatory markers following laparoscopic and open hernia repair. Surg Endosc 1995;9(6):695–8.

[33] Dunker MS, Ten Hove T, Bemelman WA, et al. Interleukin-6, C-reactive protein, and expression of human leukocyte antigen-DR on peripheral blood mononuclear cells in patients after laparoscopic vs. conventional bowel resection, a randomized study. Dis Colon Rectum 2003;46(9):1238–44.

[34] Lennard TW, Shenton BK, Borzotta A, et al. The influence of surgical operations on components of the human immune system. Br J Surg 1995;72(10):771–6.

[35] Hansbrough JF, Bender EM, Zapata-Sirvent R, et al. Altered helper and suppressor lymphocyte populations in surgical patients. A measure of postoperative immunosuppression. Am J Surg 1984;(3):303–7.

[36] Vittimberga FJ, Foley DP, Meyers WC, et al. Laparoscopic surgery and the systemic immune response. Ann Surg 1998;227(3):326–34.

[37] Ogawa K, Hirai M, Katsube T, et al. Suppression of cellular immunity by surgical stress. Surgery 2000;127(3):329–36.

[38] Hamid J, Bancewicz J, Brown R, et al. The significance of changes in blood lymphocyte populations following surgical operations. Clin Exp Immunol 1984;56(1):49–57.

[39] Decker D, Schondorf M, Bidlingmaier F, et al. Surgical stress induces a shift in the type-1/type-2 T-helper cell balance, suggesting down-regulation of cell-mediated and up-regulation of antibody-mediated immunity commensurate to the trauma. Surgery 1996; 119(3):316–25.

[40] Hensler T, Hecker H, Heeg K, et al. Distinct mechanisms of immunosuppression as a consequence of major surgery. Infect Immun 1997;65(6):2283–91.

[41] Mealy K, Gallagher H, Barry M, et al. Physiological and metabolic responses to open and laparoscopic cholecystectomy. Br J Surg 1992;79(10):1061–4.

[42] Cristaldi M, Rovati M, Elli M, et al. Lymphocytic subpopulation changes after open and laparoscopic cholecystectomy: a prospective comparative study on 38 patients. Surg Laparosc Endosc 1997;7(3):255–61.

[43] Walker CB, Bruce DM, Heys SD, et al. Minimal modulation of lymphocyte and natural killer cell subsets following minimal access surgery. Am J Surg 1999;177(1):48–54.

[44] Brune IB, Wilke W, Hensler T, et al. Downregulation of T helper type 1 immune response and altered pro-inflammatory and anti-inflammatory T cell cytokine balance following conventional but not laparoscopic surgery. Am J Surg 1999;177(1):55–60.

[45] Fujii K, Sonoda K, Izumi K, et al. T lymphocyte subsets and Th1/Th2 balance after laparoscopy-assisted distal gastrectomy. Surg Endosc 2003;17(9):1440–4.

[46] Kirman I, Cedik V, Poltaratskaia N, et al. the percentage of CD31 + T cells decreases after open but not laparoscopic surgery. Surg Endosc 2003;17(5):754–7.

[47] Bolla G, Tuzzato G. Immunologic postoperative competence after laparoscopy vs. laparotomy. Surg Endosc 2003;17:1247–50.

[48] Griffith JP, Everitt NJ, Lancaster F, et al. Influence of laparoscopic and conventional cholecystectomy upon cell-mediated immunity. Br J Surg 1995;82(5):677–80.

[49] Braga M, Vignali A, Gianotti L, et al. Laparoscopic versus open colorectal surgery, a randomized trial on short-term outcome. Ann Surg 2002;236(6):759–67.

[50] Lee SW, Southall JC, Gleason NR, et al. Time course of differences in lymphocyte proliferation rates after laparotomy vs. CO_2 insufflation. Surg Endosc 2000;14(2):145–8.

[51] Pollock RE, Lotzova E, Stanford SD. Mechanism of surgical stress impairment of human perioperative natural killer cell cytotoxicity. Arch Surg 1991;126(3):338–42.

[52] Da Costa ML, Redmond P, Bouchier-Hayes DJ. The effect of laparotomy and laparoscopy on the establishment of spontaneous tumor metastases. Surgery 1998;124(3):516–25.

[53] Da Costa ML, Redmond HP, Bouchier-Hayes DJ. Taurolidine improves survival by abrogating the accelerated development and proliferation of solid tumors and development of organ metastases from circulating tumor cells released following surgery. J Surg Res 2001;101(2):111–9.

[54] Leung KL, Tsang KS, Ng MH, et al. Lymphocyte subsets and natural killer cell cytotoxicity after laparoscopically assisted resection of rectosigmoid carcinoma. Surg Endosc 2003; 17(8):1305–10.

[55] Altamura M, Tafaro A, Casale D, et al. A comparative study between conventional and laparoscopic cholecystectomy, evaluation of phagocytic and T-cell-mediated antibacterial activities. J Clin Gastroenterol 2002;34(2):135–40.

[56] Hussein AM, Sharshira HM, Sultan MM. A comparative study between conventional and laparoscopic cholecystectomy: neutrophilic activities and cytochemical changes. Med Sci Res 1997;25:105–7.

[57] Wakefield CH, Carey PD, Foulds S, et al. Changes in major histocompatibility complex Class II expression in monocytes and T cells of patients developing infection after surgery. Br J Surg 2001;88(2):205–9.

[58] Cheadle WG, Hershman MJ, Wellhausen SR, et al. HLA-DR antigen expression on peripheral blood monocytes correlates with surgical infection. Am J Surg 1991;161(6): 639–45.

[59] Hershman MJ, Cheadle WG, Wellhausen SR, et al. Monocyte HLA-DR antigen expression characterizes clinical outcome in the trauma patient. Br J Surg 1990;77(2):204–7.

[60] Hammer JH, Nielsen HJ, Moesgaard F, et al. Duration of postoperative immunosuppression assessed by repeated delayed type hypersensitivity skin tests. Eur Surg Res 1992;24(3): 133–7.

[61] Little D, Regan M, Keane RM, et al. Perioperative immune modulation. Surgery 1993; 114(1):87–91.

[62] Pietsch JB, Meakins JL. 1976 Davis & Geck surgical essay. The delayed hypersensitivity response: clinical application in surgery. Can J Surg 1977;20(1):15–21.

[63] Christou NV, Tellado-Rodriguez J, Chartrand L, et al. Estimating mortality risk in preoperative patients using immunologic, nutritional and acute-phase response variables. Ann Surg 1989;210(1):69–77.

[64] Christou NV, Meakins JL, Gordon J, et al. The delayed hypersensitivity response and host resistance in surgical patients. 20 years later. Ann Surg 1995;222(4):534–46.

[65] Eilber FR, Morton DL. Impaired immunologic reactivity and recurrence following cancer surgery. Cancer 1970;25(2):362–7.

[66] Trokel MJ, Bessler M, Treat MR, et al. Preservation of immune response after laparoscopy. Surg Endosc 1994;8(12):1385–7.

[67] Allendorf JD, Bessler M, Whelan RL, et al. Better preservation of immune function after laparoscopic-assisted vs. open bowel resection in a murine model. Dis Colon Rectum 1996; 39(Suppl 10):S67–72.

[68] Mendoza-Sagaon M, Gitzelmann CA, Herreman-Suquet K, et al. Immune response: effects of operative stress in a pediatric model. J Pediatr Surg 1998;33(2):388–93.

[69] Gleason NR, Blanco I, Allendorf JD, et al. Delayed-type hypersensitivity response is better preserved in mice following insufflation than after laparotomy. Surg Endosc 1999;13(10): 1032–4.

[70] Mendoza-Sagaon M, Kutka MF, Talamini MA, et al. Laparoscopic Nissen fundoplication with carbon dioxide pneumoperitoneum preserves cell-mediated immunity in an immature animal model. J Pediatr Surg 2001;36(10):1564–8.

[71] Gitzelmann CA, Mendoza-Sagaon M, Talamini MA, et al. Cell-mediated immune response is better preserved by laparoscopy than laparotomy. Surgery 2000;127(1):65–71.

[72] Whelan RL, Franklin M, Holubar SD, et al. Postoperative cell mediated immune response is better preserved after laparoscopic vs open colorectal resection in humans. Surg Endosc 2003;17(6):972–8.

[73] Drysdale BE, Agarwal S, Shin HS. Macrophage-mediated tumoricidal activity: mechanisms of activation and cytotoxicity. Prog Allergy 1988;40:111–61.

[74] Redmond HP, Hofmann K, Shou J, et al. Effects of laparotomy on systemic macrophage function. Surgery 1992;111:647–55.

[75] Collet D, Vitale GC, Reynolds M, et al. Peritoneal host defenses are less impaired by laparoscopy than by open operation. Surg Endosc 1995;9(10):1059–64.

[76] Lee SW, Feingold DL, Carter JJ, et al. Peritoneal macrophage and blood monocyte functions after open and laparoscopic-assisted cecectomy in rats. Surg Endosc 2003;17(12): 1996–2002.

[77] West MA, Baker J, Bellingham J. Kinetics of decreased LPS-stimulated cytokine release by macrophages exposed to CO_2. J Surg Res 1996;63(1):269–74.

[78] Romeo C, Impellizeri P, Antonuccio P, et al. Peritoneal macrophage activity after laparoscopy or laparotomy. J Pediatr Surg 2003;38(1):97–101.

[79] Chekan EG, Nataraj C, Clary EM, et al. Intraperitoneal immunity and pneumo-peritoneum. Surg Endosc 1999;13(11):1135–8.

[80] Balague C, Targarona EM, Pujol M, et al. Peritoneal response to a septic challenge. Comparison between open laparotomy, pneumoperitoneum laparoscopy, and wall lift laparoscopy. Surg Endosc 1999;13(8):792–6.

[81] Neuhaus SJ, Watson DI, Ellis T, et al. Influence of gases on intraperitoneal immunity during laparoscopy in tumor-bearing rats. World J Surg 2000;24(10):1227–31.

[82] Watson RW, Redmond HP, McCarthy J, et al. Exposure of the peritoneal cavity to air regulates early inflammatory responses to surgery in a murine model. Br J Surg 1995;82(8): 1060–5.

[83] Jackson PG, Evans SR. Intraperitoneal macrophages and tumor immunity: a review. J Surg Oncol 2000;75(2):146–55.

[84] Kuntz C, Wunsch A, Bodeker C, et al. Effect of pressure and gas type on intraabdominal, subcutaneous and blood pH in laparoscopy. Surg Endosc 2000;14(4):367–71.

[85] West MA, Hackam DJ, Baker J, et al. Mechanism of decreased in vitro murine macrophage cytokine release after exposure to carbon dioxide: relevance to laparoscopic surgery. Ann Surg 1997;226(2):179–90.

[86] Abrams SI, Hodge JW, McLaughlin JP, et al. Adoptive immunotherapy as an in vivo model to explore antitumor mechanisms induced by a recombinant anticancer vaccine. J Immunother 1997;20:48–59.

[87] Adkins B, Charyulu V, Sun QL, et al. Early block in maturation is associated with thymic involution in mammary tumor-bearing mice. J Immunol 2000;164:5635–40.

[88] Coletta PL, Muller AM, Jones EA, et al. Lymphodepletion in the ApcMin/ + mouse model of intestinal tumorigenesis. Blood 2004;103:1050–8.

[89] Kirman I, Huang EH, Whelan RL. B cell response to tumor antigens is associated with depletion of B progenitors in murine colocarcinoma. Surgery 2004;135:313–8.

[90] Fulop G, Lee MY, Rosse C. A granulocytosis-inducing tumor inhibits the production of B lymphocytes in murine bone marrow. J Immunol 1985;135:4266–72.

[91] Shiromizu A, Suematsu T, Yamaguchi K, et al. Effect of laparotomy and laparoscopy on the establishment of lung metastasis in a murine model. Surgery 2000;128:799–805.

[92] Allendorf JD, Bessler M, Kayton ML, et al. Increased tumor establishment and growth after laparotomy vs laparoscopy in a murine model. Arch Surg 1995;130(6): 649–53.

[93] Southall JC, Lee SW, Allendorf JD, et al. Colon adenocarcinoma and B-16 melanoma grow larger following laparotomy vs. pneumoperitoneum in a murine model. Dis Colon Rectum 1998;41:564–9.

[94] Lee SW, Southall JC, Allendorf JD, et al. Tumor proliferative index is higher in mice undergoing laparotomy vs. CO_2 pneumoperitoneum. Dis Colon Rectum 1999;42: 477–81.

[95] Allendorf JD, Bessler M, Horvath KD, et al. Increased tumor establishment and growth after open vs laparoscopic bowel resection in mice. Surg Endosc 1998;12:1035–8.

[96] Lee SW, Gleason N, Blanco I, et al. Higher colon cancer tumor proliferative index and lower tumor cell death rate in mice undergoing laparotomy versus insufflation. Surg Endosc 2002;16(1):36–9.

[97] Allendorf JD, Bessler M, Horvath KD, et al. Increased tumor establishment and growth after open vs laparoscopic surgery in mice may be related to differences in postoperative T-cell function. Surg Endosc 1999;13:233–5.

[98] Davenport ML, Isley WL, Pucilowska JB, et al. Insulin-like growth factor-binding protein-3 proteolysis is induced after elective surgery. J Clin Endocrinol Metab 1992;75:590–5.

[99] Cotterill AM, Mendel P, Holly JM, et al. The differential regulation of the circulating levels of the insulin-like growth factors and their binding proteins (IGFBP) 1, 2 and 3 after elective abdominal surgery. Clin Endocrinol (oxf) 1996;44(1):91–101.

[100] Hochscheid R, Jaques G, Wegmann B. Transfection of human insulin-like growth factor-binding protein 3 gene inhibits cell growth and tumorigenicity: a cell culture model for lung cancer. J Endocrinol 2000;166:553–63.

[101] Bernard L, Babajko S, Binoux M, et al. The amino-terminal region of insulin-like growth factor binding protein-3, (1–95) IGFBP-3, induces apoptosis of MCF-7 breast carcinoma cells. Biochem Biophys Res Commun 2002;293:55–60.

[102] MacDonald RG, Schaffer BS, Kang IJ, et al. Growth inhibition and differentiation of the human colon carcinoma cell line, Caco-2, by constitutive expression of insulin-like growth factor binding protein-3. J Gastroenterol Hepatol 1999;14:72–8.

[103] Kirman I, Cekic V, Poltaratskaia N, et al. Plasma from patients undergoing major open surgery stimulates in vitro tumor growth: lower insulin-like growth factor binding protein 3 levels may, in part, account for this change. Surgery 2002;132:186–92.

[104] Kirman I, Poltoratskaia N, Sylla P, et al. Insulin-like growth factor-binding protein 3 inhibits growth of experimental colocarcinoma. Surgery 2004;136:205–9.

[105] Grimberg A. P53 and IGFBP-3: apoptosis and cancer protection. Mol Genet Metab 2000; 70:85–98.

[106] Kirman I, Poltaratskaia N, Cekic V, et al. Depletion of circulating insulin-like growth factor binding protein 3 after open surgery is associated with high interleukin-6 levels. Dis Colon Rectum 2004;47:911–7.

[107] Kirman I, Cekic V, Poltoratskaia N, et al., Open surgery induces a dramatic decrease in circulating intact IGFBP-3 in patients with colorectal cancer not seen with laparoscopic surgery. Surg Endosc 2004;Nov 11 (Epub ahead of print).

ELSEVIER
SAUNDERS

SURGICAL
CLINICS OF
NORTH AMERICA

Surg Clin N Am 85 (2005) 19–24

Laparoscopic sigmoid colectomy for diverticular disease

Anthony J. Senagore, MD, MS, MBA

Department of Colorectal Surgery, Cleveland Clinic Foundation,
9500 Euclid Ave, Desk A-30, Cleveland, OH 44195, USA

Laparoscopic colectomy (LAC) for benign and malignant lesions has become an increasingly accepted concept. There is increasingly compelling evidence that LAC does indeed provide a number of advantages, including shorter hospital stay, reduced postoperative ileus, earlier resumption of oral nutritional intake, reduced pain, and improved cosmesis [1–6]. The shortened length of stay accounts for a significant source of cost reduction, particularly in this era of nursing shortages and hospital access issues. Conversely, concerns remain regarding sources of increased cost with LAC due to the steep learning curve required, long operative procedures, and the consumption of large quantities of disposable products [7–8]. A report from the Laparoscopic Colorectal Surgery Study Group [9] demonstrated an admirably low conversion rate of 7.2%, and a low mortality rate of 1.1%. This multicenter database demonstrates the significant potential for LAC for diverticular disease. The majority of concerns related to LAC can be overcome by standardization of the surgical procedure and critical analyses regarding essential technology. This article reviews the current status of the data regarding outcomes with LAC for sigmoid diverticular disease and the author's preferred approach to the procedure.

Operative steps

A large number of studies have demonstrated the efficacy of elective laparoscopic-assisted sigmoid colectomy for diverticulitis [10–20]. The author has recently reviewed the outcomes with a large group of patients undergoing sigmoid colectomy, and the steps of the procedure will be briefly reviewed here [21]. The operative steps for LAC for the sigmoid or left colon

E-mail address: Senagoa@CCF.org

0039-6109/05/$ - see front matter © 2005 Elsevier Inc. All rights reserved.
doi:10.1016/j.suc.2004.09.007
surgical.theclinics.com

and recommended times for completion are: (1) open insertion of the umbilical port for establishment of pneumoperitoneum and peritoneal inspection (2–5 minutes); (2) placement of a 12-mm port 2 cm medial to the right anterior superior iliac spine, a 5-mm port 2 cm medial to the left anterior superior iliac spine, and a 5-mm port laterally on the right side just rostral to the umbilicus, all under direct vision with pneumoperitoneum (2–5 minutes); (3) mobilization of the mesosigmoid and mesorectum from the right side for identification of the left ureter and subsequent intracorporeal division of the vessels (10–20 minutes); (4) mobilization of the sigmoid and descending colon laterally up to the splenic flexure and medially off Gerota's fascia (10–20 minutes); (5) mobilization of the proximal rectum with division of the rectosigmoid junction with a linear endoscopic stapler (10–12 minutes); (6) division of the mesorectum at the distal resection site with control of vessels via bipolar cautery or vascular clips (15–25 minutes); (7) exteriorization of the specimen through an left lower quadrant (LLQ) muscle-splitting incision for specimen resection and anvil placement within the proximal colon (15–20 minutes); and (8) re-establishment of pneumo-peritoneum and circular-stapled anastomosis (10–15 minutes). This ap-proach allows the patient to be placed head-up for dissection of the flexure at a time when pelvic visualization has already been sacrificed, rather than changing the patient's position during the earlier dissection and losing time with each loss of exposure. If a left colectomy is required, then the head-up position can be used before making the exteriorizing incision, which will generally be a short midline at the umbilicus, rather than the LLQ review. The standardized approach to resection yields easy-to-use benchmarks for conversion, provides assurance of safe progression, and limits unnecessary equipment usage. Thaler et al [22] confirmed earlier conclusions that it is essential to perform a colorectal, not colosigmoid, anastomosis for diverticular disease to further reduce the 5% recurrence rate after surgery.

Perioperative care

In addition to standardizing the operative steps, it is important to standardize the perioperative care plans, so that optimal results can be obtained. All patients receive a mechanical bowel preparation consisting of a clear liquid diet for 24 hours preoperatively and 3 ounces of Fleets Phosphosoda (C.B. Fleet, Lynchburg, Virginia) administered the afternoon before surgery. Intravenous prophylactic cefuroxime 1 gr and metronidazole 500 mg are administered to all nonallergic patients 1 hour before the procedure. A urinary catheter is inserted at surgery and removed the following morning. The perioperative care plan includes: pre-emptive analgesia with oral diclofenac sodium (Voltaren) 50 mg the day before surgery; nasogastric tubes and drains are not employed routinely; and analgesia consists of patient-controlled epidural (bupivacaine/fentanyl) or intravenous morphine for 12 to 18 hours. All patients are offered a full liquid diet as the first meal following surgery. Thereafter, dietary intake is ad libitum, with no specific restrictions. Patients are encouraged to ambulate as soon as possible after the procedure, with a minimum of five walks outside the room the first postoperative day. The first postoperative morning patients are converted to oral analgesics, which include hydroxycodone (one or two tablets every 6 hours) and diclofenac sodium (50 mg daily). The intravenous catheters are removed the first postoperative morning unless the patient is nauseated or distended. Discharge criteria include the tolerance of three general meals without nausea or vomiting, absence of abdominal distention, adequate oral analgesia, and passage of flatus. It appears that the combination of a lesser degree of trauma with laparoscopy, early feeding, and aggressive ambulation dramatically reduces the risk of postoperative ileus and allows for early discharge after LAC. The majority of these fast-track plans can be used for open colectomy as well; however, better results occur in the laparoscopic group of patients.

Literature review

Fewer than 30% of patients who have diverticulosis will develop complications of the disease (20% diverticulits; 10% bleeding). An attack of diverticulitis can be designated as simple or complicated, based upon clinical response or more recently, computerized tomography (CT) staging. Using clinical response, simple diverticulitis (75%) responds to antibiotics, and complicated diverticulitis (25%) manifests either perforation, abscess, fistula, or obstruction [23]. More recently, Ambrosetti et al [24] have advocated CT grading, with complex defined as extraluminal air or contrast, or abscess formation. Mortality with an acute attack ranges from 1% to 5% and morbidity approaches 25%, contrasted with a 5% to 10% mortality rate and a 50% to 60% morbidity rate with a subsequent attack [25]. After an initial attack, approximately 30% of patients will have a second attack of diverticulitis, and 90% of these patients will remain symptomatic leading to resection. It is generally recommended that younger patients (<50 yrs) undergo elective resection after an initial attack; however, current data suggest that this should be restricted to patients who have severe attacks, either by CT or clinical staging, or patients who remain symptomatic after the first attack. Immunosuppressed patients should undergo surgery at the first attack, due to the high possibility of delayed recognition of complications [26].

The increasing volume of data on LAC for diverticular disease has demonstrated an acceptably low complication rate (<10%), a reduction in length of ileus (1–3 days), and a shortened length of hospitalization (2–5 days) [16–20]. The mean operative times in experienced hands have also achieved acceptable levels of 159 to 167 minutes, although conversion rates (7%–10%) are higher for this disease than for other colorectal pathologies treated by laparoscopic procedures [27–29]. Liberman et al [13] reviewed a matched control series of open and laparoscopic resections and concluded that the same benefits could be obtained with a net reduction of almost $2000 in cost. The author and colleagues [30] have recently reported on our own comparison of open and LAC for sigmoid colectomy. The data demonstrated that LAC group had a significantly shorter length of stay (3.1 versus 6.8 days), an acceptable conversion rate (6.6%), and reductions in postoperative wound (0% versus 7%) and pulmonary complications (1.6% versus 5.6%). Total direct cost per case was significantly less for LAC ($3458 ± $437 versus $4321 ± $501). Two additional cohort studies confirmed similar findings of significantly lower costs and a shortened length of stay with laparoscopic management of diverticular disease [31,32].

It is clear, however, that complicated diverticular disease does present additional challenges, and should not be undertaken without considerable experience in LAC. The German multicenter study group [9] identified a doubling of morbidity with complicated (29%) versus noncomplicated (15%) diverticultis and a significantly higher conversion rate. Similar findings were reported by the Texas Endosurgery Institute, with higher conversion rates and complications in perforated or fistulous disease [33]; however, as surgeons gain more experience, single-stage resection and repair of colovesical fistulas from diverticular disease can be managed effectively with acceptable morbidity and conversion rates [34]. Of some concern, however, is the use of laparoscopic colorrhaphy coupled with abscess drainage for complicated diverticulitis. This has been advocated by Da Rold and coauthors [35], who employed this technique in 7 patients who have no apparent complications. It is unclear if these patients could have been managed either by imaged guided drainage or with single-stage resection. Incomplete management of the septic focus may be problematic.

Summary

Laparoscopic management of sigmoid diverticular disease has emerged as an important adjunct to the armamentarium of surgical options for this disease process. Although there are no prospective randomized studies directly comparing laparoscopic and open colectomy for diverticulitis, the comparative studies provide compelling data. The magnitude of the benefits achieved with laparoscopic colectomy in the hands of experienced laparoscopic colon surgeons may soon be sufficient to make LAC the standard of care.

References

[1] Chen HH, Wexner SD, Weiss EG, et al. Laparoscopic colectomy for benign colorectal disease is associated with as a significant reduction in disability compared with laparotomy. Surg Endosc 1998;12(12):1397–400.

[2] Ballantyne GH. Laparoscopic-assisted colorectal surgery: review of results in 752 patients. Gastroenterologist 1995;3:75–89.

[3] Bruce CJ, Coller JA, Murray JJ, et al. Laparoscopic resection for diverticular disease. Dis Colon Rectum 1996;39(Suppl 10):S1–6.

[4] Carbajo CM, Martin del Olmo JC, Blanco JI, et al. The laparoscopic approach in the treatment of diverticular colon disease. J Society of Laparoendoscopic Surgeons 1998;2: 159–61.

[5] Senagore AJ, Kilbride MJ, Luchtefeld MA, et al. Superior nitrogen balance after laparoscopic-assisted colectomy. Ann Surg 1995;221:171–5.

[6] Fleshman JW, Nelson H, Peters WR, et al. Early results of laparoscopic surgery for colorectal cancer. Retrospective analysis of 372 patients treated by Clinical Outcomes of Surgical Therapy (COST) Study Group. Dis Colon Rectum 1996;39(Suppl, 10):S53–8.

[7] Schlachta CM, Mamazza J, Seshadri PA, et al. Defining a learning curve for laparoscopic colorectal resections. Dis Colon Rectum 2001;44:217–22.

[8] Marusch F, Gastinger I, Schnieder C, et al. Kockerling F and the Laparoscopic Colorectal Study Group (LCSSG). Importance of conversion for results obtained with laparoscopic colorectal surgery. Dis Colon Rectum 2001;44:207–16.

[9] Kockerling F, Schneider C, Reymond MA, et al. Laparoscopic resection of sigmoid diverticulitis. Results of a multicenter study. Laparaoscopic Colorectal Surgery Study Group. Surg Endosc 1999;13(6):567–71.

[10] Bouvet M, Mansfield PF, Skibber KM, et al. Clinical, pathologic and economic parameters of laparoscopic colon resection for cancer. American Journal of Surgery 1998;176(6):554–8.

[11] Bergamaschi R, Arnaud JP. Immediately recognizable benefits and drawbacks after laparoscopic resection for benign disease. Surg Endosc 1997;11(8):802–4.

[12] Senagore AJ, Luchtefeld MA, Mackeigan JM, et al. Open colectomy vs. laparoscopic colectomy: are there differences? Am Surg 1993;59:549–54.

[13] Liberman MA, Phillips BJ, Carroll M, et al. Laparoscopic colectomy vs traditional colectomy for diverticulitis. Surg Endosc 1996;10:15–8.

[14] Wexner SD, Reissman P, Pfeifer J, et al. Laparoscopic colorectal surgery: analysis of 140 cases. Surg Endosc 1996;10:133–6.

[15] Agachan F, Joo JS, Weiss EG, et al. Intraoperative laparoscopic complications: are we getting better? Dis Colon Rectum 1996;39(Suppl 10):S14–9.

[16] Sher ME, Agachan F, Bortul M, et al. Laparoscopic surgery for diverticulitis. Surg Endosc 1997;11(3):264–7.

[17] Falk PM, Beart RW Jr, Wexner SD, et al. Laparoscopic colectomy: a critical appraisal. Dis Colon Rectum 1993;36:28–34.

[18] Lumley JW, Fielding GA, Rhodes M, et al. Laparoscopic-assisted colorectal surgery. Lessons learned from 240 consecutive patients. Dis Colon Rectum 1996;39:155–9.

[19] Pfeifer J, Wexner SD, Reissman P, et al. Laparoscopic vs open colon surgery. Costs and outcome. Surg Endosc 1995;9:1322–6.

[20] Saba AK, Kerlakian GM, Kasper GC, et al. Laparoscopic assisted colectomies versus open colectomy. J Laparoendosc Surg 1995;5:1–6.

[21] Senagore AJ, Duepree HJ, Delaney CP, et al. Results of a standardized technique and postoperative care plan for laparoscopic sigmoid colectomy: a 30 month experience. Dis Colon Rectum 2003;46(4):503–9.

[22] Thaler K, Baig MK, Berho M, et al. Determinants of recurrence after sigmoid resection for uncomplicated diverticulitis. Dis Colon Retum 2003;46(11):1572–3.

[23] Young-Fadok TM, Pemberton JH. Colonic diverticular disease: epidemiology and pathophysiology. In: Rose BD, editor. UpToDate in medicine (CD_ROM). Wellesly (MA): UpToDate; 2000.

[24] Ambrosetti P, Jenny A, Becker C, et al. Acute left colonic diverticulitis—compared performance of computed tomography and water soluble contrast enema: prospective evaluation of 420 patients. Dis Colon Rectum 2000;43(10):1363–7.

[25] Sarin S, Boulos PB. Long term outcome of patients presenting with acute complications of diverticular disease. Ann R Coll Surg Engl 1994;76:117–20.

[26] Perkins JD, Shield CF III, Chang FC, et al. Acute diverticulitis:comparison of treatment in immunocompromised and non-immunocompromised patients. Am J Surg 1984;148:745–8.

[27] Muckleroy SK, Ratzer ER, Fenoglio ME. Laparoscopic colon surgery for benign disease: a comparison to open surgery. JSLS 1999;3:33–7.

[28] Schlachta CM, Mamazza J, Poulin EC. Laparoscopic sigmoid resection for acute and chronic diverticulitis. An outcomes comparison with laparoscopic resection for non-diverticular disease. Surg Endosc 1999;13:649–53.

[29] Schwandner O, Farke S, Fischer F, et al. Laparoscopic colectomy for recurrent and complicated diverticulitis: a prospective study of 396 patients. Langenbecks Arch Surg 2004; 389(2):97–103.

[30] Senagore AJ, Duepree HJ, Delaney CP, et al. Cost structure of laparoscopic and open sigmoid colectomy for diverticular disease: similarities and differences. Dis Colon Rectum 2002;45(4):485–90.

[31] Dwivedi A, Chahin F, Agrawal S, et al. Laparoscopic colectomy vs open colectomy for sigmoid diverticular disease. Dis Colon Rectum 2002;45(10):1309–14.

[32] Lawrence DM, Paasquale MD, Wasser TE. Laparoscopic versus open sigmoid colectomy for diverticulitis. Am Surg 2003;69:499–503.

[33] Franklin ME, Norman JP, Jacobs M, et al. Is laparoscopic surgery applicable to complicated colonic diverticular disease? Surg Endosc 1997;11(10):1021–5.

[34] Menenakos E, Hahnloser D, Nassiopoulos K, et al. Laparoscopic surgery for fistulas that complicate diverticular disease. Langebecks Arch Surg 2003;388(3):189–93.

[35] Da Rold AR, Guerriero S, Fiamingo P, et al. Laparoscopic colorrhaphy, irrigation and drainage in the treatment of complicated acute diverticulitis: initial experience. Chir Ital 2004;56(1):95–8.

ELSEVIER
SAUNDERS

Surg Clin N Am 85 (2005) 25–34

SURGICAL
CLINICS OF
NORTH AMERICA

Laparoscopic surgery in the treatment of Crohn's disease

Jeffrey W. Milsom, MD

Section of Colorectal Surgery, New York Presbyterian Hospital, Weill Medical College of Cornell University, 525 East 68th Street, New York, NY 10021, USA

Crohn's disease (CD) is one of the most challenging arenas of intestinal surgery. Many of its pathologic features, such as intense inflammation, a thickened mesentery, enteric fistulae, and skip areas of intestinal involvement, have justifiably deterred surgeons from considering a laparoscopic approach in the surgical therapy of CD. Nonetheless, most patients who have CD understand that they have a high (70%–90%) probability of needing surgery at some point; thus they are extremely motivated to undergo an operation that could involve minimal scarring and a faster recovery.

This article presents the current evidence for the use of laparoscopic techniques in the surgical therapy of Crohn's disease of the small and large intestine. Sections outlining indications and some key aspects of our current laparoscopic techniques to manage Crohn's disease are also included.

Methods

Search of literature

The literature data bases MEDLINE, EMBASE, and the Cochrane Central Controlled Trials Register were searched for randomized controlled trials for the years 1991 to 2004. The MeSh-terms _colon* >, _colectomy >, _proctectomy* >, _intestine-large >, _intestine-small >, _colonic Crohn's >, _rectal Crohn's >, _anal Crohn's >, _laparoscopy* >, and _laparoscopic surgery* > were used for the search, and over 200 publications were found. Clinical studies that contained only patients who had other diseases were excluded from further analysis, as were publications

---

E-mail address: jwm2001@med.cornell.edu

that gave only laboratory data without any clinical outcome. Clinical studies that included patients who had other diseases were evaluated, but studies reported in multiple publications or data given only in abstracts were also excluded from the analysis. Laparoscopic, laparoscopic-assisted, and hand-assisted procedures or resections were included. Interestingly, there is only one prospective randomized trial currently available in the literature using the above criteria [1] The author attempted to evaluate the evidence available in the literature using a process for systematic weighting of level and grading of evidence established by the American College of Chest Physicians [2,3].

Outcome measures

The following short-term outcome measures were analyzed: duration of surgery, estimated intraoperative blood loss, functional data (postoperative pulmonary function, duration of postoperative ileus), postoperative hospital stay, morbidity (total, surgical, general), and mortality.

Whenever available, long-term data on recurrence of disease and duration of follow-up were extracted from the publications.

Review of the literature

Although a number of clinical reports have described that laparoscopic assisted ileocolic resections are feasible and safe in the treatment of Crohn's disease, most have been uncontrolled and nonrandomized [4–12]. Additionally, there are reports that question whether or not there are any advantages at all in the use of laparoscopic methods compared with conventional methods in Crohn's disease [13]. In a recent study, our surgical group at the Cleveland Clinic showed in a prospective randomized trial that there were advantages to laparoscopic methods compared with open methods in the recovery of patients who had ileocolic CD [1]. Details of this trial, as well as other clinical trials on surgery for Crohn's disease (comparative and descriptive, arbitrarily including only those with more than 20 laparoscopic cases) published in the past 5 years, are summarized in Tables 1 and 2 [1,4–6,13–19].

Surgical therapies/technical considerations

Indications/contraindications for a laparoscopic approach in Crohn's disease surgery

The indications for surgical therapy should not differ between open (conventional) and laparoscopic surgery:

- Severe obstructive or septic complications
- Significant hemorrhage

Table 1
Characteristics of clinical trials on Crohn's disease surgery using laparoscopic methods

Study	Method	#Patients	Disease site	Outcomes
Milsom 2001 [1]	RCT	60 (31 L, 29, O)	IC	MST: pulm function; other: op time, analgesic dose, duration of ileus, morbidity, hospital stay
Huilgol 2004 [14]	Comp	40 (21,19)	IC	Similar
Bergamaschi 2003 [15]	Comp	92 (39,53)	IC	Similar, also long term SBO
Shore 2003 [16]	Comp	40 (20,20)	IC	Similar, also costs
Benoist 2003 [13]	Comp	56 (24,32)	IC	Similar
Von Allmen 2003 [17]	Comp	28 (12,16)	IC	Similar, pediatric pts
Duepree 2002 [19]	Comp	45 (21,24)	IC	Similar, also costs
Luan 2000 [18]	Comp	47 (24,23)	Mixed	Similar
Hasegawa 2003 [6]	Descr	52	IC	Feasibility, LOS, complications
Hamel 2002 [5]	Descr	41	IC	Similar
Evans 2002 [4]	Descr	84	IC	Similar

Abbreviations: Comp, comparative; Descr, descriptive study of only laparoscopic surgery patients; IC, ileocolic disease; L, laparoscopic; LOS, length of hospital stay; mixed, mixture of small- and large-bowel surgery patients; MST, main study criterion; O, open contemporaneous trial; RCT, randomized controlled trial; SBO, small bowel obstruction rate.

- Fulminant inflammation not controlled by medication
- Intolerable side effects due to the treatment, including growth retardation in pediatric patients

Contraindications to laparoscopic surgery include

- Diffuse peritonitis
- Acute obstruction with distension accompanied by dilated loops of intestine
- History of multiple previous laparotomies, known dense intra-abdominal adhesions
- Coagulopathy not correctable at time of operation
- Portal hypertension with known intra-abdominal varices

The use of laparoscopic techniques in CD may be divided into three categories: (1) diagnostic laparoscopy, (2) Diversion techniques (eg, ileostomy or colostomy), and (3) resectional therapies.

The last category includes: (1) "pure" laparoscopic techniques, in which only small incisions are used throughout the operation, and the specimen is removed at the end of the operation; (2) "laparoscopic-assisted" techniques, in which some portion of the operation (eg, the anastomosis) is done through a limited incision; and (3) "hand-assisted" techniques, in which a limited incision is made permitting the surgeon's hand to be used during

Table 2
Outcome measures following laparoscopic or conventional surgery for the treatment of Crohn's disease

Study	Operating time (mins)	Conversion (%)	Complications	Analgesics	Bowel function	LOS (days)	Other
Milsom 2001 [1]	L 70>O	7	L < O	NS	NS	L 1 d	PFTs: L adv
Huigol 2004 [14]	NS	–	NS	NS	L adv	L adv	–
Bergamaschi 2003 [15]	L 80>O	–	NS	–	–	L adv 5 d	L: dec SBO 5 y
Shore 2003 [16]	NS	–	NS	–	L adv 2 d	L adv 4 d	L cost <O
Benoist 2003 [13]	NS	17	O < L	NS	NS	NS	–
Von Allmen 2003 [17]	–	–	–	L < O	L adv 2 d	L adv 6 d	Pediatric patients
Dupree 2002 [19]	–	4	NS	–	L adv 2 d	L adv 2 d	Cost L sl < O
Luan 2000 [18]	–	29	NS	L < O	L adv 3 d	L adv 3 d	EBL L < O
Hasegawa 2003 [6]	–	16	–	–	–	–	Safe, feasible, incl rec. CD and fistulas
Hamel 2002 [5]	–	26	–	–	–	–	Similar
Evans 2002 [4]	–	18	–	–	–	–	Feasible in patients with recurrence, abscess, fistula

Abbreviations: adv, advantage; d, days; EBL, estimated blood loss; L, laparoscopic group; LOS, length of stay; NS, no statistical difference; O, open group; PFTs, pulmonary function tests; rec, recurrent; SBO, small bowel obstruction; sl, slightly.

the laparoscopic portion of the operation, done in concert with use of laparoscopic tools.

Diagnostic laparoscopy

Our group considers a diagnostic laparoscopy for Crohn's disease to be important in certain rare circumstances. When a patient has an unusual presentation of his disease (ie, terminal ileitis not responding to the conventional medical therapy over a relatively short time period), or if a patient has poorly explained abdominal pains with an otherwise negative work-up, it may behoove the medical-surgical team to consider a diagnostic laparoscopy in the evaluation of a patient, especially before potent immune-suppressing drugs are given over a prolonged period. An example of this may be the patient who has ileitis and who is febrile, who is unresponsive to medical treatments including antibiotics, and whose CT scan shows evidence of mesenteric lymphadenopathy. The ruling out of another disease such as lymphoma may be important in such a patient, and diagnostic laparoscopy may be an expeditious means of obtaining a biopsy and treating the patient appropriately.

Diversion techniques

When a CD patient has severe unremitting sepsis related to anorectal Crohn's, with or without abscess, there may be a consideration for a diversion (ie, ileostomy). Often, this is a prelude to more definitive local therapy, even proctectomy, but in the short term, a laparoscopic loop ileostomy may bridge the patient to a better state of physical and mental health so as to permit further definitive treatment.

The method generally employs only two or three puncture sites on the abdominal wall, including the stoma site, and can be done fairly expeditiously. Anorectal sepsis can be treated at the same operative session if needed.

Resectional therapies

Pure laparoscopic treatment of both small- and large-bowel diseases is not commonly described in the literature. There were no articles in the literature in which a pure technique was obviously used in performing laparoscopic bowel resections. Thus the vast majority of procedures are either laparoscopic-assisted or hand-assisted laparoscopic surgery (HALS) procedures. The rationale for this has been that an incision somewhere on the abdominal wall is needed, whether done by a pure method or by an assisted method, and the size of this incision is nearly the same whichever technique is used. Thus the handling of the thickened Crohn's mesentery and intestine is much easier when an assisted method is used. Likewise, although there is no evidence in the literature to support the HALS method over other methods, it appears to offer advantages in instances in which the disease leads to marked inflammation and adherence to surrounding soft tissues. In these instances, hand dissection may permit the surgeon to accomplish a procedure in which the only significant incision is placed in the suprapubic area, where it will likely be barely visible.

The technique of resectional therapies has been described in many articles. Basically, when our group performs this surgery for ileocolic CD, there are usually four or five cannulas placed, including in the area of the umbilicus and in the four quadrants lateral to the rectus sheath. Consideration should be given to the prospect that the patient may need an ileostomy sometime in his life, so incisions should be kept away from these areas. When HALS is considered, we begin with a 7 to 7.5 cm suprapubic incision about two finger breadths above the symphysis pubis, using a classical Pfannenstiel incision that preserves (splits) the rectus muscles after making a transverse incision through the anterior sheath. A port is then placed (GelPort Device, Applied Medical, Rancho Santa Margarita, California) into this incision, and other ports, starting with the umbilical one, are placed with hand assistance.

Some special technical considerations

Each case starts with a diagnostic laparoscopy. During every laparoscopic procedure, regardless of type, the initial phase of the operation should be a diagnostic study. Our group emphasizes that a thorough exploration of all intra-abdominal structures should be undertaken, including the ovaries, Fallopian tubes, and uterus in females. The entire small bowel should be "run," starting at the ligament of Treitz to the end of the small bowel, especially because small-bowel radiograph series notoriously miss strictures in patients undergoing surgery for CD. A suture marking the most proximal extent of disease is often useful later in the operation when the diseased intestine is drawn out of the limited abdominal incision for removal or repair.

Handling the mesentery

The thickened mesentery of CD can be challenging to divide even during open surgery. In nearly all cases, our group uses a Ligasure device (ValleyLab, Boulder, Colorado), either 10 mm (Ligasure Atlas) or 5 mm (Ligasure V), which can be used in vessels up to 7 mm in diameter. It is effective when used properly for nearly any type of mesentery, although there is a technique to its use that is important in effectively ligating vessels, mainly involving slow clamping and cutting of the tissue.

Perspective

Now that 13 years have elapsed since the first reported colonic resections using laparoscopic methods (mainly done for colonic malignancies), there are certainly many reported clinical experiences of laparoscopic surgical therapy for both large- and small-bowel Crohn's disease. These include pure laparoscopic techniques, laparoscopic-assisted methods, and use of HALS surgery. Also included in these techniques are both diversions and resectional therapies. Although the literature is not sparse, there remains only one randomized controlled trial (RCT) comparing a laparoscopic-assisted method with open surgery in the treatment of ileocolonic CD.

Conclusions

The results of this systematic review provide primarily level 3 or 4 evidence for the use of laparoscopic techniques in Crohn's disease surgery. Considering these prerequisites, short-term significant benefits of laparoscopic compared with conventional colorectal resection have been demonstrated for intraoperative blood loss, pulmonary function, duration of postoperative ileus, and hospital stay. The rather small but significant improvement of pulmonary function after laparoscopic compared with conventional surgery and the faster postoperative recovery of pulmonary function may be reflected in a slightly lower incidence of pulmonary complications after laparoscopic colorectal resections. The only disadvantage of laparoscopic surgery, an increased operative time of approximately 40 minutes, is significant, and may also be economically relevant.

Because of the reduced size of incisions in laparoscopic colorectal surgery, the reduction of surgical complications, especially wound infections, could have been anticipated.

Although the incidence of mechanical bowel obstruction caused by intraperitoneal adhesions has not been addressed in any RCTs so far in colorectal surgery, Winslow et al did not detect a difference in the incidence of incisional hernia in their RCT for colorectal cancer that included only 83 patients [20]. Therefore, these nononcological long term-results of laparoscopic versus conventional colorectal surgery have to be further investigated in RCTs.

Finally, no trials of any kind with adequate sample size provide any data on long-term outcomes. In summary, there is currently level 3 or 4 evidence, primarily from descriptive studies, that short- and long-term results of laparoscopic colorectal surgery for Crohn's disease may be superior to results achieved by conventional resection, leading to a grade B or C level of recommendation for using the laparoscopic approach in the surgical treatment of Crohn's disease.

Discussion

In conclusion, a systematic review of the literature to identify randomized controlled or other clinical trials comparing short-term and long-term outcomes of laparoscopic or conventional resections and diversions in the treatment of Crohn's disease showed some benefits of the laparoscopic technique:

- Improved postoperative pulmonary function
- Slight reduction in duration of postoperative ileus
- Decreased hospital stay
- A slight decrease of the cost of direct hospital costs for laparoscopic surgery
- A moderate decrease of surgical morbidity

Perioperative treatment of both groups was traditional in almost all trials, however. Modern multimodal concepts of perioperative treatment may improve the postoperative course regardless of the type of access to the abdominal cavity used.

Long-term outcomes (eg, disease recurrence, complications such as adhesive obstructions and hernias) after curative laparoscopic or conventional resection of Crohn's disease cannot be assessed with adequate accuracy, because there are no results from large multicenter trials. New multicenter RCTs comparing differences between laparoscopic and conventional colorectal surgery are needed, but will probably not come to fruition in the near future, owing to the fact that many patients now seek this technique from specialized centers, and the outcomes, at least cosmetically, are extremely appealing to these patients. Future studies should also address outcomes between laparoscopic versus open Crohn's surgery, to include the use of hand-assisted methods.

Some final questions to consider, based on the currently available data in the literature

- Does the laparoscopic approach really lead to less morbidity? When traditional perioperative treatment with systemic opiod analgesia, postoperative nonfeeding strategy, and delayed mobilization is performed, laparoscopic resection of small bowel and large bowel Crohn's may decrease local as well as general morbidity.
- Does the laparoscopic approach lead to less mortality? There are no data to support the assumption that laparoscopic resection of small bowel and colorectal Crohn's will decrease postoperative mortality.
- Has the laparoscopic approach led to any short-term advantages? Under traditional perioperative treatment, the laparoscopic treatment probably results in less pain, less analgesic consumption, better pulmonary function, and a shorter duration of postoperative ileus. It remains unclear, however, whether this will still hold true when a perioperative multimodal treatment is used.
- Does the laparoscopic approach increase hospital costs? To date, no RCTs have addressed cost savings for the hospital or society (recovery period after the hospitalization) if patients are treated laparoscopically.

Operative time is increased in laparoscopic surgery, however, and this may increase costs caused by the operation itself.

- Are the long-term results in favor of the laparoscopic approach? The outcomes for laparoscopic and conventional resection of ileocolic and large-bowel Crohn's do not seem to be different. It has been hypothesized that the laparoscopic approach may reduce the long-term-incidence of hernia, intraperitoneal adhesions, and reoperations for mechanical ileus; however, there are no data of any type available yet to support or contradict this hypothesis.
- Will there be further technological breakthroughs or improvements in the laparoscopic or minimally invasive methods that may widen the differences between laparoscopic methods and conventional ones? This is very speculative, but there will almost certainly be further technological advances that will improve the outcomes of patients undergoing laparoscopic surgery as well as conventional surgery.

References

[1] Milsom JW, Hammerhofer KA, Boehm B, et al. A prospective randomized trial comparing laparoscopic versus conventional surgery in refractory ileocolic Crohn's disease. Dis Colon Rectum 2001;44(1):1–19.

[2] Cook DL, Guyatt GH, Laupacis A, et al. Rules of evidence and clinical recommendations on the use of antithrombotic agents. Chest 1992;102(Suppl 4):305–311S.

[3] Sackett DL. Rules of evidence and clinical recommendations on the use of anti-thrombotic agents. Chest 1989;95(Suppl 2):2–4S.

[4] Evans J, Poritz L, MacRae H. Influence of experience on laparoscopic ileocolic resection for Crohn's disease. Dis Colon Rectum 2002;45:1595–600.

[5] Hamel CT, Pikarsky AJ, Wexner SD. Laparoscopically assisted hemicolectomy for Crohn's disease: are we still getting better? Am Surg 2002;68:83–6.

[6] Hasegawa H, Watanabe M, Nishibori H, et al. Laparoscopic surgery for recurrent Crohn's disease. Br J Surg 2003;90:970–3.

[7] Bauer JJ, Harris MT, Grumbach NM, et al. Laparoscopic-assisted intestinal resection for Crohn's disease. Which patients are good candidates? J Clin Gastroenterol 1996;23:44–6.

[8] Ludwig KA, Milsom JW, Church JM, et al. Preliminary experience with laparoscopic intestinal surgery for Crohn's disease. Am J Surg 1996;171:52–5.

[9] Wu JS, Birnbaum EH, Kodner IJ, et al. Laparoscopic-assisted ileocolic resections in patients with Crohn's disease: are abscesses, phlegmons, or recurrent disease contraindications? Surgery 1997;122:682–9.

[10] Lui CD, Rolandelli R, Ashley SW, et al. Laparoscopic surgery for inflammatory bowel disease. Am Surg 1995;61:1054–6.

[11] Reissman P, Salky BA, Pfeifer J, et al. Laparoscopic surgery in the management of inflammatory bowel disease. Am J Surg 1996;171:47–51.

[12] Ogunbiyi OA, Fleshman JW. Place of laparoscopic surgery in Crohn's disease. Baillieres Clin Gastroenterol 1998;12:157–65.

[13] Benoist S, Panis Y, Beaufour A, et al. Laparoscopic ileocecal resection in Crohn's disease: a case matched comparison with open resection. Surg Endosc 2003;17:814–8.

[14] Huilgol RL, Wright CM, Solomon MJ. Laparoscopic versus open ileocolic resection for Crohn's disease. J Laparoendosc Adv Surg Tech A 2004;14:61–5.

[15] Bergamaschi R, Pessaux P, Arnaud JP. Comparison of conventional and laparoscopic ileocolic resection for Crohn's disease. Dis Colon Rectum 2003;46:1129–33.

[16] Shore G, Gonzalez QH, Bondora A, et al. Laparoscopic vs. conventional ileocolectomy for primary Crohn's disease. Arch Surg 2003;138:76–9.

[17] von Allmen D, Markowitz JE, York A, et al. Laparoscopic-assisted bowel resection offers advantages over open surgery for treated segmental Crohn's disease in children. J Pediatr Surg 2003;38:963–5.

[18] Luan X, Gross E. Laparoscopic assisted surgery for Crohn's disease: an initial experience and results. J Tongji Med Univ 2000;20:332–5.

[19] Duepree HJ, Senagore AJ, Delaney CP, et al. Advantages of laparoscopic resection for ileocecal Crohn's disease. Dis Colon Rectum 2002;45:605–10.

[20] Winslow ER, Fleshman JW, Birnbaum EH, et al. Wound complications of laparoscopic vs open colectomy. Surg Endosc 2002;16:1420–5.

ELSEVIER
SAUNDERS

SURGICAL
CLINICS OF
NORTH AMERICA

Surg Clin N Am 85 (2005) 35–47

Laparoscopic surgery for ulcerative colitis

Steven D. Wexner, MD, FACS, FRCS,
FRCS (Ed)[a,b,c,*], Susan M. Cera, MD[a]

[a]Department of Colorectal Surgery, Cleveland Clinic Florida,
2950 Cleveland Clinic Boulevard, Weston, FL 33331, USA
[b]Department of Surgery, Ohio State University Health Sciences Center at the
Cleveland Clinic Foundation, 260 Meiling Hall, 370 West 9th Avenue,
Columbus, OH 43210-1238, USA
[c]Department of Surgery, University of South Florida College of Medicine,
12901 Bruce B. Downs Boulevard, Tampa, FL 33612, USA

Laparoscopic techniques have revolutionized the management of many colorectal diseases. Virtually every procedure has been attempted laparoscopically. Success lies in the documented claims of shorter hospitalization, faster recovery, and improved cosmesis. The application of laparoscopy for some disease processes has required acquisition of experience and an evolution of technique to optimize benefit. Inflammatory diseases of the intestine, such as Crohn's disease, ulcerative colitis, and diverticulitis, have proven particularly challenging to the laparoscopic surgeon because of the technical demands posed by their complicating inflammatory nature. Early laparoscopic experience involved long operative times, high rates of conversion, and excessive operating room costs, which raised concern about the physiologic and economic advantages. Over the last decade, intense investigation and subsequent refinements in technique and technology have led to considerable advances and a clearly established role for laparoscopic management of Crohn's disease and diverticulitis; however, laparoscopy for ulcerative colitis has not proven to be as promising.

Laparoscopic procedures described for ulcerative colitis include laparoscopic subtotal colectomy, total proctocolectomy, and restorative proctocolectomy. These procedures involve laparoscopic mobilization of long segments of large bowel, control of multiple and variable blood vessels,

* Corresponding author.
E-mail address: wexners@ccf.org (S.D. Wexner).

0039-6109/05/$ - see front matter © 2005 Elsevier Inc. All rights reserved.
doi:10.1016/j.suc.2004.09.009
surgical.theclinics.com

experience in laparoscopic access of both flexures, and advanced techniques for specimen extraction and ileal pouch creation. Mobilization of the rectum with laparoscopic assistance is especially difficult and time-consuming. These maneuvers require a significant learning curve that must be mastered to confer benefit. Although numerous experienced laparoscopic teams have documented their ability to complete these procedures, persistently long operative times and proportionately elevated rates of morbidity in some studies appear to counter the advantages. Despite focus on variations in technique and improvements in technology over the last decade, the benefits of minimized physiologic impact and shortened recovery have been realized in only a few studies of experienced surgeons. The question remains as to the universal application and appropriateness of these procedures in the surgical management of ulcerative colitis. Indications for these procedures remain controversial.

From the beginning

The earliest reports of the laparoscopic approach to ulcerative colitis are from the early 1990s. Peters [1] first reported the technique of laparoscopic proctocolectomy for two patients who had ulcerative colitis. Subsequently, Wexner et al [2] published the first case-controlled report on the outcome of laparoscopic-assisted total colectomy with ileoproctostomy or ileoanal reservoir in five patients who had ulcerative colitis, familial adenomatous polyposis, and colonic inertia, and who were compared with a matched group undergoing the open procedure. The laparoscopic-assisted group demonstrated significantly longer operative time (234 versus 145 minutes). Postoperative ileus and hospital length of stay were not statistically significant. The cosmetically superior incision was 35% smaller compared with the incision length of the laparotomy group, but the authors suspected that the significant amount of traction needed to accomplish the procedure through this incision was the reason no improvement in ileus duration was noted in the laparoscopic group. Consequently, the length of stay did not differ significantly between the two groups, averaging 8.0 days for the laparoscopic group and 9.2 days for the open group. No major morbidity occurred in either group, but no immediately recognizable patient benefits were identified.

Enthusiasm for the laparoscopic approach for ulcerative colitis was further tempered after publication of a 1994 study by this same group [3]. Twenty-two patients who underwent laparoscopic-assisted restorative proctocolectomy, the majority of whom had ulcerative colitis, were compared with 20 patients matched for age, gender, and diagnosis undergoing the open procedure. The mean operative time for the laparoscopic group was significantly longer than for the open group (240 versus 120 minutes), the postoperative morbidity was higher (55% versus 30%), and the transfusion requirement significantly greater (73% versus 35%). No differences were identified in resolution of ileus

(4.2 versus 3.3 days) or the mean length of hospital stay (8.7 versus 8.9 days). At the conclusion of this study, the authors discouraged the use of minimally invasive techniques for patients requiring restorative proctocolectomy in absence of the theoretical advantages seen with other laparoscopic procedures.

Retrospective case studies

Since then, numerous surgical groups have reported their outcome of laparoscopy in the treatment of ulcerative colitis (Tables 1,2). Because of technical variations, instrument availability, differences in amount of laparoscopic dissection performed, and influence of the learning curve and training, comparison of laparoscopic versus conventional techniques among institutions is difficult. In addition, the majority of reported outcomes are based on retrospective analyses in absence of a control group. No prospective, randomized trials exist to date. Consequently, outcomes of the laparoscopic approach are reported with significant variability, although several trends have become apparent over the past decade. Numerous experienced laparoscopic teams have documented the ability to complete laparoscopic procedures for ulcerative colitis, but persistently long operative times (up to 8 hours) and proportionately elevated rates of morbidity (0%–60%) appear to counter the advantages (see Table 1). In 1995, Liu and associates [4] reported on a group of patients undergoing laparoscopic-assisted colectomies for inflammatory bowel disease. Five of the 10 patients had ulcerative colitis and underwent laparoscopic-assisted total abdominal colectomies with ileal pouch reservoirs. The remaining patients underwent

Table 1
Retrospective studies on procedures for ulcerative colitis

Author	Year	n	OR time	Morbidity	Conversion	LOS
Tucker [27]	1995	4	5 h 27 min	6%	13.2%	6
Rhodes [28]	1994	5	5 h 2 min	60%	-	-
Liu [3]	1995	5	8 h	20%	20% (1/5)	7
Thibault [5]	1995	4	7 h 18 min	-	-	10
Reissman [10]	1996	30	3 h 30 min	30%	10%	6.5
Santoro [6]	1999	5	6 h 4 min	20%	0	12.6
Pace[a] [7]	2002	13	4 h 25 min	46%	8%	7
Hasegawa [29]	2002	18	6 h	33.3%	0	9
Ky [24]	2002	32	5 h 15 min	34%	0	6
Kienle[b] [8]	2003	59	5 h 20 min	18.6%	5/59 (8.5%)	15
Range			(5 h 30 min–8 h)	(0%–60%)	(0%–20%)	(6%–12.6)

Abbreviations: LOS, length of stay; OR, operating room.
[a] All patients underwent laparoscopic completion proctectomy with ileal pouch reservoir.
[b] Included procedures for ulcerative colitis and familial adenomatous polyposis.

Table 2
Comparative studies of laparoscopic versus open procedures for ulcerative colitis

Author	Year	Lap/open		OR Time	Conversion	Morbidity	LOS
Wexner [2]	1992	Lap	5	3 h 30 min	0	0%	8.0
		Open	5	2 h 30 min	-	0%	9.2
Schmitt [3]	1994	Lap	22	4 h	0	68%	8.7
		Open	20	2 h	-	35%	8.9
Marcello [16]	2000	Lap	20	5 h 30 min	0	20%	7
		Open	20	3 h 45 min	-	25%	8
Araki[a] [17]	2001	Lap	21	3 h 35 min	-	33.3%	3.6
		Open	11	3 h 18 min	-	45.5%	3.9
Dunker [19]	2001	Lap	16	4 h 52 min	0	12.5%	9.9
		Open	17	2 h 39 min	-	23.5%	12.5
Hashimoto[b] [18]	2001	Lap	11	8 h 23 min	0	63.6%	24.1
		Open	13	7 h 2 min	-	38.4%	31.3

Data in bold type reflect statistically significant differences in comparisons.

Abbreviations: FAP, familial adenomatous polyposis; Lap, laparoscopic; LOS, length of stay; OR, operating room; UC, ulcerative colitis.

[a] Included patients who underwent laparoscopic or open total abdominal colectomy with ileorectal anastomosis.

[b] FAP and UC patients included.

operations for complications of Crohn's disease, including segmental colectomies. Despite mixing the data from the laparoscopic procedures for both Crohn's and ulcerative colitis, operative times were high (8 hours) and only a trend was noted toward shorter hospital stay. The morbidity and conversion rates were both 20%. The authors concluded that the only advantages included excellent cosmetic results and a theoretical reduction in adhesions for patients who have inflammatory bowel disease, and who physiologically cannot afford future intestinal resections.

In 1995, Thibault and Poulin [5] published their preliminary results of complete intracorporeal total proctocolectomy. Using a laparoscopic-assisted technique, the mean operative time was 7 hours and 18 minutes, with an average blood loss of 500 to 800 cc and a mean hospital stay of 10 days. Given these initial results, the authors modified their initial techniques to a laparoscopic-assisted approach, decreasing their operative time to 4 hours. They also noted a decrease in their hospital stay to 8.3 days. Variations in the amount of surgery performed laparoscopically appeared to have minimal effect on the length of surgery and length of stay.

In 1999, Santoro and coauthors [6] also included a completely intra-corporeal dissection and vascular division, thereby avoiding the excessive traction that Wexner et al claimed to be responsible for the prolonged postoperative ileus and narcotic requirements. They reported on five pa-tients, of whom three had ulcerative colitis, who underwent laparoscopic-assisted restorative proctocolectomy. Excessively long operative times (480 minutes for the first case) associated with their purely laparoscopic technique offset the possible benefits of reduced postoperative ileus. Consequently, the average length of stay was prolonged, at an average of 12.6 days, longer than seen with Wexner et al, with a morbidity rate of 20%, larger than seen with Wexner et al. With experience, operative time decreased significantly to 240 minutes in their later cases.

Laparoscopic restorative proctectomy in patients who have already undergone subtotal colectomy requires a long operative time. In 2002, Pace and coauthors [7] studied 13 patients who underwent laparoscopic completion proctectomy with creation of an ileal reservoir. The median operative time was 6 hours 15 minutes, with one conversion, a morbidity rate of 46%, and a mean length of stay of 7 days. A quality-of-life survey revealed no differences from studies of patients undergoing the open procedure. Isolated laparoscopic mobilization of the rectum has proven to be time-consuming. The authors concluded that although the procedure was technically feasible in experienced centers, the technique required further evolution, because no obvious benefits were apparent from this study.

In 2003, Kienle and colleagues [8] reported on nine patients who underwent laparoscopic-assisted restorative proctocolectomy in a prospective, cohort study. Five conversions occurred, all of them in patients who had an elevated body mass index (BMI). The authors concluded that an elevated BMI prohibited laparoscopic success, and that failure of the laparoscopic technique was associated with major complications. Good patient selection was obviously a critical factor in successful completion of this extensive procedure.

Comparative studies of laparoscopic procedures for ulcerative colitis and Crohn's disease

Earlier in the decade, during the developmental years of laparoscopic colorectal surgery, patients' demands for laparoscopy increased, new instrumentation was being introduced, and surgeons were gaining more experience. Laparoscopic segmental resections rapidly transitioned into widespread practice, because of immediate and obvious benefits. Laparoscopy was being applied to other inflammatory disorders of the intestine, including Crohn's disease, with much success. Compared with laparotomy, documented benefits of laparoscopic-assisted ileocolic resection for Crohn's disease included better cosmesis, lower incidence of laparotomy for postoperative bowel obstruction, a 50% decrease in recovery time, more rapid return to social and sexual interaction, and decreased costs [9]. Laparoscopic ileocolic resection and laparoscopic segmental small-bowel resections and strictureplasties became well-established procedures because of the feasibility, safety, and beneficial postoperative outcomes noted.

In a 1996 study from Cleveland Clinic Florida [10], the results of 72 consecutive cases of inflammatory bowel disease were managed with the laparoscopic approach. Twenty-two of these patients underwent laparoscopic total proctocolectomy with ileal reservoir for ulcerative colitis, 2 patients underwent total colectomy with ileostomy for ulcerative colitis, and 6 patients underwent total colectomy with ileorectal anastomosis for Crohn's disease. These cases were compared with a selection of patients undergoing various other procedures for Crohn's disease, the most common of which was ileocolic resection for terminal ileitis (n = 30). When compared with ileocolic resection, total colectomy was associated with longer operative time (210 minutes versus 150 minutes), longer hospital stay (8.7 versus 5.2 days), and higher rate of morbidity (30% versus 10%). The versatility, feasibility, and safety of laparoscopic procedures for Crohn's disease were demonstrated, whereas excessive operative times and threefold higher morbidity of laparoscopic-assisted total colectomy proved prohibitive. Thus, the former procedures were endorsed and the latter procedure was not advocated for routine use.

In a 1998 publication from Cleveland Clinic Florida [11], a review of the literature from 1992 to 1997 revealed that patients who had terminal ileitis or anal Crohn's disease requiring fecal diversion enjoyed many advantages conferred from the laparoscopic approach, including decreased pain, length of hospitalization, and disability, along with improved cosmesis and a reduction in symptomatic postoperative adhesive disease. These benefits were achieved with no increase in morbidity or expense. Conversely, the analysis revealed that the use of laparoscopic technology for restorative proctocolectomy for ulcerative colitis was associated with a longer operative time and an increased incidence of both intraoperative and postoperative complications compared with laparotomy. In addition to a review of the literature, the report included an evaluation of 28 restorative proctocolectomies compared with a matched group of patients who underwent standard laparotomy. The laparoscopic-assisted group demonstrated much longer operative times (240 minutes versus 140 minutes), required blood transfusion in twice as many patients, and had greater postoperative morbidity (43% versus 30%). This report re-emphasized that laparoscopy was advantageous for the surgical management of Crohn's disease, but not routinely justified for the treatment of ulcerative colitis. The differences in outcome were explained by the differences in the procedures. Ileocolic resection, segmental bowel resection, stoma creation, and stricturoplasty are well-suited for laparoscopic-assisted surgery. Total colectomy is a much lengthier and technically difficult procedure, because of the need for extensive mobilization of bowel and rectum and the creation of the ileal reservoir.

Although there are no comparative studies involving patients undergoing laparoscopic restorative proctocolectomies for ulcerative colitis and those undergoing laparoscopic surgery for sigmoid diverticulitis, studies involving laparoscopic sigmoid resection have demonstrated many benefits of the minimally invasive approach for those who have diverticulitis. Benefits noted in all age groups include less intraoperative blood loss, less postoperative pain, shortened postoperative ileus, shorter hospitalization, earlier return to work, improved cosmesis, reduced disability, and reduction of postoperative adhesions [12–15]. The morbidity rates of laparoscopic sigmoid resection are equivalent or superior to those rates noted in well-matched patients after laparotomy. Laparoscopy has found an important role in the surgical management of sigmoid diverticulitis.

Comparative studies of laparoscopic versus open procedures for ulcerative colitis

Only a few controlled studies regarding laparoscopy for the treatment of ulcerative colitis have been reported. The controlled studies have been performed at highly experienced institutions and provide the most convincing data with regard to the differences between the laparoscopic and open approaches of surgery for ulcerative colitis. In 2000, a study by Marcello and coworkers [16] from the Cleveland Clinic Foundation was published involving surgeons who performed more than 700 laparoscopic colorectal procedures in 6 years, more than 100 of which were total abdominal colectomies. Twenty consecutive patients (13 mucosal ulcerative colitis (MUC), 7 familial adenomatous polyposis (FAP)) undergoing laparoscopic total proctocolectomy with ileal J-pouch were compared with 20 matched patients undergoing the conventional procedure [3]. The median length of operating room time was 100 minutes longer for the laparoscopic group (330 versus 225 minutes). The estimated blood loss and postoperative complication rates were the same and no conversions were required. The length of stay was shortened by 1 day in the laparoscopic group (7 versus 8 days). In the hands of skilled laparoscopic surgeons, the issue of increased morbidity seen in earlier studies was eliminated. Selection bias secondary to careful patient selection may or may not have played a role; however, the advantages of a 1-day shorter hospital stay and improved cosmesis occurred even with a highly skilled team and a decade of experience.

Outcomes from the remainder of the case-controlled studies are listed in Table 2. Only one study by Araki and colleagues [17] demonstrated no statistical significance in operative times between the laparoscopic and open approach (3 hours, 35 minutes versus 3 hours, 18 minutes, respectively). This may be partly explained by the technique used, because only colonic mobilization was performed laparoscopically, whereas vessel transection and rectal mobilization were performed through a minilaparotomy incision. The remainder of the studies, however, except for that of Marcello's group [16], employed this same technique, with significantly longer operative times in the laparoscopic group (overall average 4 hours, 55 minutes for laparoscopic versus 2 hours, 10 minutes for open). The technique employed in the study involved laparoscopic colonic and rectal mobilization, with intracorporeal vessel transection reserving the minilaparotomy incision for specimen extraction [16]. Although their operative times were longer in the laparoscopic group (5 hours, 30 minutes versus 3 hours, 45 minutes), they were within the range reported for the alternate technique used in the other studies.

Over the past decade, morbidity rates in these comparative studies have improved, and have been found to be equivalent with the open procedure in all studies except one. This study by Hashimoto and coworkers [18] involved a hand-sewn rectal mucosectomy as part of the laparoscopic-assisted procedures. The morbidity rate in the laparoscopic group was 60% higher than in the open group, but consisted mainly of postoperative bowel obstructions and wound infections. In addition, of the studies performed at highly experienced institutions, none reported any conversions, implying improvement in expertise with experience.

Finally, most of these comparative studies also reveal shortened hospital lengths of stay in comparing laparoscopic versus open groups [16,18,19]. The study by Araki and coauthors [17] showed equivalent length of stay between the two groups (3.6 versus 3.9 days, laparoscopic versus open), but both groups had much shorter stays compared with the earlier experience at the beginning of the decade, in which the length of stay for both and laparoscopic procedures averaged 8 to 9 days.

Some surgeons have justified the prolonged operative times of the laparoscopic approach with significantly improved cosmesis. In fact, the cosmetic benefit alone has been shown to be of paramount importance to patients, because many undergoing this procedure are young and have great concern with body image. Dunker et al [19] performed a comparative study to assess the impact of cosmesis as well as functional outcome and quality of life. Sixteen patients who underwent laparoscopic-assisted total proctocolectomy were compared with 19 patients who underwent conventional surgery. No differences were identified between the two groups with respect to functional outcome as measured by the number of stools during the day and night, stool consistency (solid, semisolid, liquid), soiling, incontinence, need for antidiarrheal medication, dietary restrictions, sexual activity, and sexual satisfaction. In addition, no differences were identified with regard to quality of life, as assessed by physical functioning, role limitations, bodily pain, general health, vitality, social limitations, emotional role limitations, and mental functioning. Satisfaction with the cosmetic result of the scar was significantly higher with the laparoscopic group; however, body image scores between the two groups were not significantly different. Conclusions drawn from this study included that functional outcome and quality of life did not differ from conventional ileal pouch anal anastomosis (IPAA). In addition, better cosmesis was the most important long-term advantage of the laparoscopic approach. Dunker and a different group of coauthors [20] also demonstrated the importance of patient cosmesis in a previous study with regard to ileocolic resection for Crohn's disease. Because of concern for body image and self-confidence, patients' responses to a questionnaire included preferences to undergo the laparoscopic versus the open approach, even in the face of hypothetical increase risk of ureteral injury and excess out-of-pocket expenses.

Significant controversy continues with regard to the optimal technique, the extent of laparoscopically performed dissection, use of stoma, and risk-benefit analysis for the patient. No individual center has gleaned enough experience with all the various techniques; therefore, significant short-comings exist because of this nonrandomized approach. Consensus and standardization are also needed with respect to data collection, definition of complications and conversion, and quality-of-life assessment. Data from properly controlled and adequately powered randomized studies are lacking for many laparoscopic procedures, except for Crohn's disease, in which a recent study by Milsom and coauthors [21] demonstrated improved pulmonary function, earlier return of bowel function, and decreased length of postoperative stay. Only in the hands of experienced surgeons with careful patient selection have decreased morbidity and shortened hospital stay been realized. The role of laparoscopic total colectomy' in the future surgical armamentarium is pending prospective, randomized trials. In addition, future efforts should be directed toward optimizing patient selection, surgeon training, surgical techniques to minimize morbidity and maximize satisfactory outcomes, and developing instruments and tools to shorten operative times for laparoscopic colorectal surgery procedures.

The role of laparoscopy in acute ulcerative colitis

Reports of the use of laparoscopy in urgent procedures for ulcerative colitis have had mixed results (Table 3). Bell and Seymour [22] reported on 18 patients who had fulminant ulcerative colitis and who were treated with laparoscopic-assisted restorative proctocolectomy. This subset of patients is particularly challenged by immunologic, nutritional, and inflammatory derangements imposed by both the disease and its treatment. Postoperative complications occurred in 33%, but a significantly decreased length of stay (5.0 versus 8.8 days) was noted when compared with 6 patients who underwent the open procedure for the same indication. The study authors concluded that the high morbidity rate was related to their compromised status at the time of surgery, given their aggressive colitis and high-dose immunosuppressive therapy. They also concluded that the recovery time was much decreased compared with the open group, thereby substantiating

Table 3
Total colectomy for acute colitis

Author	Year	Lap/open	Mean OR time	Conversion
Marcello [23][a]	2001	Lap 19	210	0%
		Open 29	120	-
Bell [22][b]	2002	Lap 18	220–360	0%
		Open 6	-	-

Abbreviations: Lap, laparoscopic; OR, operating room.
[a] Nonfulminant colitis.
[b] Fulminant colitis.

this approach as an alternative to the conventional treatment of fulminant colitis.

In 2001, Marcello et al [23] published their results of laparoscopic-assisted total abdominal colectomy in patients who had acute but not fulminant ulcerative colitis and Crohn's disease requiring urgent colectomy. The report included the experience of 19 laparoscopic and 29 conventional total colectomies with end ileostomy and buried mucous fistula. No conversions or intraoperative colostomies occurred in the laparoscopic group. The laparoscopic group demonstrated longer operative times (210 versus 120 minutes) but comparative blood loss (100 cc), earlier return of bowel function (1 versus 2 days), and shorter hospital stay (4 versus 6 days). Complications occurred in 3 (16%) of the laparoscopic patients and in 7 (24%) of the conventional patients. The study's authors concluded that laparoscopic total colectomy is feasible and safe in patients who have acute nonfulminant colitis, and may lead to faster recovery than conventional surgery in the hands of an experienced team.

The role of laparoscopy in obviating the need for diverting ileostomy—the outcome of one-stage procedures

The controversy regarding whether the minimally invasive laparoscopic approach to restorative proctocolectomy allows for the safe omission of a diverting ileostomy is not resolved. In a prospective cohort study by Kienle and associates [8], only 9 out of 59 patients undergoing laparoscopic-assisted restorative proctocolectomy were given a diverting ileostomy at the primary procedure if the dissection was difficult or the anastomosis was felt to be under tension. Nine patients, all of whom were on either high-dose immunosuppresssants or had an elevated BMI, required secondary ileostomies. The authors of the study concluded that the minimally invasive approach does not reduce the need for a protective ileostomy in selected patients, but that the omission or addition of an ileostomy remains to be defined. In contrast, Ky and colleagues [24] performed a single-stage laparoscopic restorative proctocolectomy on 32 patients, only one of whom had a pouch leak that required a secondary ileostomy. The authors of the study concluded this to be a safe procedure and that it avoids the risk of a second operation, the inconvenience of a second hospital admission, and the cost of a second procedure. In Dunker et al's study [19], 10 of 15 patients undergoing the laparoscopic procedure were not given an ileostomy, without any complication related to this omission. Single-stage procedures may be safe when performed by experienced surgeons in a select group of patients.

The role of minilaparotomy and handoscopy in ulcerative colitis

Minilaparotomy has been documented as an alternative to laparoscopy for the minimally invasive approach, and offers some advantages over laparoscopy for ulcerative colitis. Brown and coworkers [25] reported the surgical and postoperative outcomes of 13 patients who underwent open restorative proctocolectomy using an minilaparotomy Pfannensteil incision (14 cm) in comparison to a group of 12 undergoing the laparoscopic-assisted procedure (wound length 8.5 cm). The procedure is performed with the assistance of a lighted St. Mark's retractor for mobilization of the colon. The mean operative time was significantly shorter, and other parameters, including duration of analgesia pump, first ileostomy function, length of ileus, and length of hospital stay, were no different. Cosmesis was maintained and all other parameters were equivalent to the open procedure. The only advantage of a laparoscopic-assisted procedure over a minilaparotomy technique was the size of the wound. Development of better wound retractors and lighting systems may facilitate popularity of the minilaparotomy technique for ulcerative colitis.

Handoscopy or hand-assisted laparoscopic surgery (HALS) may also prove to be another alternative to laparoscopy for ulcerative colitis. Though no studies of this technique for restorative proctocolectomy have been published to date, restorative proctocolectomy is a suitable operation, because a minilaparotomy incision is required for extraction of the large intestine and completion of the surgery. This operation would avoid the major morbidity of laparotomy by using the advantages of laparoscopy during the initial dissection stage. HALS offers the ability to do more complex operations by offering tactile feedback, safer traction and counter-traction on tissues, and the benefit of digital blunt dissection. Completion of the procedure through a minilaparotomy incision allows application of standard surgical instruments and extraction of the specimen. Although HALS has proven beneficial in other colorectal procedures, outcome with respect to procedures for ulcerative colitis await publication of comparative studies.

Summary

After a decade of experience and improvements in technology, several factors remain barriers to the widespread practice of laparoscopic total colectomy for ulcerative colitis. These procedures have a steep leaning curve and require a level of expertise that is difficult to acquire outside a colorectal institution that specializes in laparoscopy and inflammatory bowel disease. For most surgeons with limited training in laparoscopy for inflammatory disorders, the technical demands of laparoscopic total colectomy may lend to higher morbidity, conversion rates, and cost, as seen with the earlier studies of laparoscopic total colectomy. With experience, the higher morbidity and increased rates of blood transfusion requirements noted in early reports have virtually been eliminated, and replaced by shortened hospital length of stay; however, prolonged operative times continue to offset the advantages by posing a barrier in institutions with a high workload of cases and where operating room time is at a premium. For these surgeons, additional operating time (as high as 8 hours in some series) may be an unacceptable disadvantage, even if other surgical parameters are unchanged. Other surgeons have justified these prolonged procedures by claiming significantly improved cosmesis, postoperative recovery, and decreased future risk of postoperative adhesive disease. The importance of cosmesis to patients should not be underestimated. In addition, shortened recovery is also of extreme importance in those young patients who have chronic disease, malnourishment, and sustained immunosuppression, and who are most likely to benefit from a minimally invasive approach. Finally, decreased postoperative adhesive disease has recently been confirmed in a report on long-term outcomes of laparoscopic procedures in which a decreased rate of subsequent reoperations secondary to ventral hernia repair and small-bowel obstruction was noted, implying additional advantages for these patients who have long life expectancy [26].

As with any area of medicine, appropriate critical analysis of a technology is needed for widespread acceptance. Although several studies, including a randomized, prospective report, have demonstrated the benefits of laparoscopy in the surgical management of Crohn's disease [10,11,21], the lack of reports from prospective, randomized, case-controlled studies of laparoscopy for ulcerative colitis prevents the proclamation of conclusive, demonstrable benefits.

References

[1] Peters WR. Laparoscopic total proctocolectomy with creation of ileostomy for ulcerative colitis: report of two cases. J Laparoendosc Surg 1992;2:175.
[2] Wexner SD, Johansen OB, Nogueras JJ, et al. Laparoscopic total abdominal colectomy: a prospective trial. Dis Colon Rectum 1992;35:651–5.
[3] Schmitt SL, Cohen SM, Wexner SD, et al. Does laparoscopic-assisted ileal pouch anal anastomosis reduce the length of hospitalization? Int J Colorect Dis 1994;9:134–7.
[4] Liu CD, Rolandelli R, Ashley SW, et al. Laparoscopic surgery for inflammatory bowel disease. Am Surg 1995;61:1054–6.
[5] Thibault C, Poulin EC. Total laparoscopic proctocolectomy and laparoscopic-assisted proctocolectomy for inflammatory bowel disease: operative technique and preliminary report. Surg Laparosc Endosc 1995;5:472–6.
[6] Santoro E, Carlini M, Carboni F, et al. Laparoscopic total proctocolectomy with ileal J-pouch anastomosis. Hepatogastroenterology 1999;46:894–9.
[7] Pace DE, Seshadri PA, Chiasson PM, et al. Early experience with laparoscopic ileal pouch-anal anastomosis for ulcerative colitis. Surg Laparosc Endosc 2002;12(5):337–41.
[8] Kienle P, Weitz J, Benner A, et al. Laparoscopically assisted colectomy and ileoanal pouch procedure with and without protective ileostomy. Surg Endosc 2003;17:716–20.
[9] Joo JS, Agachan F, Wexner SD. Laparoscopic surgery for lower GI fistulas. Surg Endosc 1997;11(2):116–8.
[10] Reissman P, Salky BA, Pfeifer J, et al. Laparoscopic surgery in the management of inflammatory bowel disease. Am J Surg 1996;171(1):47–51.
[11] Sardinha TC, Wexner SD. Laparoscopy for inflammatory bowel disease: pros and cons. World J Surg 1998;22(4):370–4.

[12] Liberman MA, Phillips EH, Carroll BJ, et al. Laparoscopic colectomy versus traditional colectomy for diverticulitis outcome and costs. Surg Endosc 1996;10:15–8.

[13] Kholer L, Rixen D, Troidl H. Laparoscopic colorectal resection for diverticulitis. Int J Colorectal Dis 1998;13:43–7.

[14] Dwivedi A, Chahin F, Agrawal S, et al. Laparoscopic colectomy versus open colectomy for sigmoid diverticular disease. Dis Colon Rectum 2002;45(10):1309–14.

[15] Senagore AJ, Duepree HJ, Delaney CP, et al. Cost structure of laparoscopic and open sigmoid colectomy for diverticular disease: similarities and differences. Dis Colon Rectum 2002;45(4):485–90.

[16] Marcello PW, Milsom JW, Wong SK, et al. Laparoscopic restorative proctocolectomy: a case-matched comparative study with open restorative proctocolectomy. Dis Colon Rectum 2000;43:604–8.

[17] Araki Y, Ishibashi N, Ogata Y, et al. The usefulness of restorative laparoscopic-assisted total colectomy for ulcerative colitis. Kurume Med J 2001;48:99–103.

[18] Hashimoto A, Funayama Y, Naito H, et al. Laparoscopic-assisted versus conventional restorative proctocolectomy with rectal mucosectomy. Surg Today 2001;31(3):210–4.

[19] Dunker MS, Bemelman WA, Slors JFM, et al. Functional outcome, quality of life, body image, and cosmesis in patients after assisted-assisted and conventional restorative proctocolectomy: a comparative study. Dis Colon Rectum 2001;44:1800–7.

[20] Dunker MS, Stiggelbout AM, van Hogezand RA, et al. Cosmesis and body image after laparoscopic-assisted and open ileocolic resection for Crohn's disease. Surg Endosc 1998; 12(11):1334–40.

[21] Milsom JW, Hammerhofer KA, Bohm B, et al. Prospective, randomized trial comparing laparoscopic versus conventional surgery for refractory ileocolic Crohn's disease. Dis Colon Rect 2001;44(1):1–8.

[22] Bell RL, Seymour NE. Laparoscopic treatment of fulminant colitis. Surg Endosc 2002; 16:1778–82.

[23] Marcello PW, Milsom JW, Wong SK, et al. Laparoscopic total colectomy for acute colitis: a case controlled study. Dis Colon Rectum 2001;44:1441–5.

[24] Ky AJ, Sonoda T, Milsom JW. One-stage laparoscopic restorative proctocolectomy: an alternative to the conventional approach? Dis Colon Rectum 2002;45:207–11.

[25] Brown SR, Eu KW, Seon-Choen F. Consecutive series of laparoscopic-assisted versus minilaparotomy restorative proctocolectomies. Dis Colon Rectum 2001;44(3):397–400.

[26] Duepree HJ, Senagore AJ, Delaney CP. Does means of access affect the incidence of small bowel obstruction and ventral hernia after bowel resection? Laparoscopy versus laparotomy. J Am Coll Surg 2003;197(2):177–81.

[27] Tucker JG, Ambroze WL, Orangio GR, et al. Laparoscopically assisted bowel surgery: Analysis of 114 cases. Surg Endosc 1995;9:297–300.

[28] Rhodes M, Stitz RW. Laparoscopic subtotal colectomy. Seminars in Colon and Rectal Surgery 1994;5(4):267–70.

[29] Hasegawa H, Wantanabe M, Baba H, et al. Laparoscopic restorative proctocolectomy for patients with ulcerative colitis. J Laparoendosc Adv Surg Tech A 2002;12(6):403–6.

ELSEVIER
SAUNDERS

SURGICAL
CLINICS OF
NORTH AMERICA

Surg Clin N Am 85 (2005) 49–60

Laparoscopic surgery for colon cancer

P.A. Paraskeva, BSc (Hons), MBBS (Hons), PhD,
FRCS, O. Aziz, BSc (Hons), MBBS, MRCS,
A. Darzi, MD, FRCS, FACS, FRCSI*

*Department of Surgical Oncology and Technology, Imperial College London, 10th Floor,
QEQM Wing, St. Mary's Hospital, London W2 1NY, England*

Successful laparoscopic surgical techniques have been well described for benign conditions such as gallbladder disease and hiatus hernia. The application of these approaches to malignant disease has been approached with skepticism following initial reports of wound metastases occurring in laparoscopic procedures for a variety of different indications [1–13]. Surgeons re-examined the role of laparoscopic surgery for many surgically treated malignancies such as colorectal carcinoma [14]. The potential advantages of laparoscopic assisted surgery for major organ surgery have been well documented, with a decreased hospital stay, less postoperative pain, and quicker return to normal function. It is the cancer patient, however, who stands to potentially benefit more from a minimally invasive approach, due to the decreased surgical trauma and less immune function disruption. The decreased immune paresis should allow less tumor recurrence and improve patient survival as well as quality of life [15–16]. Despite these obvious benefits, acceptance of the laparoscopic approach for malignant disease has been gradual. It is a technically more challenging surgical procedure; could this, with other environmental factors, represent a compromise in oncological safety?

Of vital importance during the evolution of the laparoscopic approach to colonic surgery have been the effects of training, skill of the surgeon, and technical aspects during the procedure that affect the outcome of the patient. This article focuses on the techniques for colonic resection, followed by an examination of the potential patient and health care benefits of laparoscopic surgery. Finally, the authors examine the outcomes of minimally invasive surgery in colon cancer patients.

* Corresponding author.
E-mail address: a.darzi@imperial.ac.uk (A. Darzi).

0039-6109/05/$ - see front matter © 2005 Elsevier Inc. All rights reserved.
doi:10.1016/j.suc.2004.09.001

Laparoscopic colectomy—operative technique

Early problems during laparoscopic colectomy necessitating conversion were related to poor instrumentation; however, innovations by surgeons and industry have led to increased technical feasibility. Most colonic tumors are amenable to excision, unless they are fixed due to local spread. The addition of hand-related devices has also led to increased accessibility for colorectal procedures. These make logical sense, because a larger incision is required to remove the specimen, which can be capitalized upon for the procedure itself.

The importance of adhering to sound oncological principles during either open or laparoscopic surgery, such as no-touch technique and the en bloc resection of the primary tumor and any other structures involved locally, together with the lymphatics and vascular structures, should never be forgotten. Laparoscopy lacks the manual dexterity afforded by open surgery, which may give rise to some theoretical problems—inappropriate handling of the tumor, especially by the inexperienced, for example. Differences in surgical technique or skill may account for the great variability in outcome from colorectal cancer among surgeons in terms of morbidity, local control, and survival.

Indications to guide surgeons wishing to undertake laparoscopic colectomy were provided by Smith. This study used laparoscopic right and left hemicolectomies as benchmark procedures. It reported that to become an accomplished laparoscopic surgeon would require performing at least 15 laparoscopic colectomies; the average surgeon would, however, have to perform at least 25 hand-assisted cases and 50 totally laparoscopic cases [17]. The mean operating times in this study were 130 minutes for accomplished surgeons. Earlier series demonstrated learning curve effects with operative time up to a mean of 240 minutes [18].

An adaptation of the laparoscopic approach in which a hand-assist device is inserted into the abdomen has been shown to be effective in some patients. A prospective randomized multicenter trial compared hand-assisted and standard laparoscopic colectomy [19]. The study found that parameters such as operative time, length of abdominal incision, return of bowel function, and hospital stay were comparable between the two techniques. The authors of the study concluded that hand-assisted laparoscopic surgery retained all the benefits of the standard laparoscopic approach, with the convenience of a hand to aid during surgery. Because the patient requires an abdominal incision for specimen removal in both approaches, the use of a hand-assist device seem to make good sense. It would also seem from further studies using hand assisted approaches to laparoscopic colectomies [20–25] that the conversion rate to open is lower than in a totally laparoscopic approach, and may also aid surgeons in the initial part of their learning curves.

Clinical evidence

The institution of the laparoscopic approach to curative resection of malignant growths has been controversial. After the widespread acceptance of laparoscopic cholecystectomy, the application of minimally invasive surgery for cancer seemed a natural progression. There is no doubt that the laparoscopic approach is feasible; the oncological safety of performing these procedures has, however, been questioned. This doubt has caused many surgeons to abandon or not subscribe to a minimally invasive approach for cancer surgery. The majority of work relating to laparoscopic resection has been in the area of colorectal resection, mainly due to nature of the disease; hence the majority of the further discussion in this paper will therefore be related to this.

Laparoscopic curative resection applied to procedures such as gastrectomy and adrenalectomy has also been described. Initial evidence for laparoscopic resections focused mainly on the technical aspects of the procedure. Indiscriminate use of laparoscopic techniques outside carefully controlled trials led to confusing results that were difficult to draw significant conclusions from.

Since the first laparoscopic colonic resection for malignancy in 1991 [26], many researchers have reported initial series and commented on problems with technical delivery of the procedure, lengthy operating times, high conversion rates, and the worry over adequacy of excision and iatrogenic dissemination of tumor [27–31]. Due to the resulting increasing concerns, surgeons developed a more selective policy with their patients, which acted as prelude to randomized controlled trials.

Potential advantages of the laparoscopic approach

Gastrointestinal motility

An obvious advantage of the laparoscopic approach for the cancer patient is the reduction of the postoperative ileus. These patients may already be nutritionally depleted and are at increased risk of thromboembolic disease; both of these factors are adversely affected by a postoperative ileus. In their early experience with laparoscopic-assisted abdomino-peringal (AP) resection, Darzi et al demonstrated that ileus time as measured by time to passage of flatus was reduced [32]. The phenomenon may be related to factors associated with the approach and the reduction in pain [33–37] when compared with open surgery, and hence the decreased requirements for analgesia, and also to the reduction in handling of the bowel and the use of a closed operative environment. As studies on the postoperative management of laparoscopic surgery cannot be blinded, this raises the question of whether these patients are positively discriminated to by the managing surgeon. This makes conclusions difficult to reach from existing data, although earlier feeding and a faster recovery have been demonstrated [38]. More objective data of recovery of ileus comes from Schwenk and colleagues, who showed faster colonic transit of radio-opaque markers in a laparoscopic colectomy group when compared with an open surgery group [39].

Larger randomized studies have given clearer evidence of benefit of the laparoscopic approach. Milsom and coworkers compared a small group of laparoscopic-assisted and conventional colectomies, and investigated time to flatus when both groups were managed with the same postoperative feeding regimen [40]. It was shown that the laparoscopic group passed flatus earlier than the open group. A further study by Lacy and associates again examined similar questions with slightly larger numbers of patients, and found that the laparoscopic group had the advantage in time to flatus [41]. Table 1 summarizes results from randomized studies.

Quality of life costs

Minimally invasive technique practitioners advocate that they can lead to faster patient recovery, and hence lower health service costs and increased quality of life, when compared with open procedures [44,45]. The cost savings proposed by the laparoscopic approach, however, can be quickly absorbed by technology costs and theater consumables; moreover, subsequently converting laparoscopic patients to open surgery can increase health costs. Various studies have investigated health costs. Bokey and coauthors looked at the cost of laparoscopic right hemicolectomy and found it to be greater when compared with that of open surgery. Their study revealed that most of the costs were theater-related. This study, however, did not measure the positive effect an earlier return to activity from a laparoscopic approach would have to the economy in general [46].

It is obvious that quality of life has many component parameters that can be measured; most studies have focused on postoperative pain. The assessment of postoperative pain is a parameter that logically should improve with a minimally invasive approach. In reality, however, many trials are immediately biased by different management by surgical teams. Typically, as laparoscopic cases are often allowed to eat earlier then traditional cases, regular oral analgesia is often used, thereby causing an

Table 1
Randomized trials investigating return of bowel function after laparoscopic colectomy

Authors	Year	No. of patients	Time to bowels open	Significantly shorter than open
Milsom [40]	1998	54	3	Yes
Curet [42]	2000	18	2.7	Yes
Lacy [41]	2002	111	1.5	Yes
Hasegawa [43]	2003	29	2	Yes

apparent decrease in the usage of parenteral analgesics. Randomized trials in which some of theses variables have been controlled have shown that there are definite benefits to postoperative pain in the laparoscopic group on day 1; however, in subsequent days, there are no significant differences in postoperative pain between laparoscopic and open groups [47].

Weeks et al [47] looked more broadly at quality of life issues, investigating patients preoperatively, at 2 days, 2 weeks, and 2 months postoperative. Interestingly, they again demonstrated an initial analgesic advantage in the laparoscopic group when compared with open; however, other quality of life parameters we not significantly different. Twenty-five percent of patients who were converted from a laparoscopic to an open approach reported consistently lower quality of life scores when compared with those who underwent the standard laparoscopic approach. Recently Nelson and coworkers [48] reported on a large group of patients who underwent laparoscopic colectomy. They demonstrated a significantly lower parenteral analgesic requirement, and to a lesser degree, a lower oral analgesic requirement in the laparoscopic group when compared with the open group. Table 2 summarizes results from randomized studies.

Length of hospital stay

The topic of effect of the minimally invasive approach on length of hospital stay after colectomy is commonly investigated. This is understandable, because one of the major potential economical advantages of laparoscopy is to decrease hospital costs in this fashion. Many trials exist, giving a wide variety of data. Retrospective and prospective studies have shown ranges from 5 days to 16 days in hospital [49–54]. Randomized trials in the main support the view that a laparoscopic-assisted colectomy results in a shorter time in the hospital [33]. Interestingly however, Milsom showed no difference in length of stay between laparoscopic and open groups [40]. One of the reasons for this may be that because the study was also investigating return of bowel function, patients in both arms of the trial were allowed to eat only on day 3 postoperatively. This may have inhibited the progress of members of the laparoscopic group, who may have been able to eat on day 1 post surgery. Despite this, there is good evidence that having

Table 2
Randomized trials investigating reduction in pain after laparoscopic colectomy

Author	Year	No. of patients	Less pain	Significantly less pain than open
Stage [52]	1997	15	Yes	Yes
Schwenk [53]	1998	30	Yes	Yes
Milsom [40]	1998	54	Yes	Yes
Weeks [47]	2002	168	Yes	Yes
Hasegawa [43]	2003	29	Yes	Yes
Nelson [48]	2004	345	Yes	Yes

a laparoscopic-assisted colectomy has significant advantages in decreasing hospital stay. Recently, Nelson and colleagues reported on a larger group of patients and showed a definite significant decrease in hospitalization [48]. Table 3 summarizes results from randomized trials.

Adequacy of excision and lymph node harvest

One of the initial major concerns of the laparoscopic approach for curative cancer resection was that it could lead to a breach of well-established oncological principles. Inadequate resection margins, poor lymph node harvest, and port-site metastases put the laparoscopic excision of colorectal carcinoma in jeopardy. Since these early experiences, many studies have demonstrated adequate excision margins and lymph node harvest [55–58].

Vascular ligation with regards to the tumor specimen is another issue under controversy. Common sense dictates that the higher the vascular pedicle taken with the specimen, the less likely the recurrence [59]. Corder and collaborators, however, studied a series of 143 consecutive patients using a proportional hazards analysis and found no differences in recurrence or mortality, compared with the method of vascular ligation [60]. There are those, however, who believe that high ligation is useful for the reduction in the incidence of port-site metastasis [61] that can be safely undertaken laparoscopically.

Long-term outcomes and survival—evidence from trials

When evaluating laparoscopic surgery and comparing it with the open approach, complications, morbidity and mortality, oncological safety, and achievement of proposed benefits are the most important parameters to consider. In 1994, Wexner and Cohen further investigated the feasibility of laparoscopic colectomy; however, on review of the literature at the time, they reported the overall incidence of post-site metastases as 4% [62]. In 1997, Bonjer et al further reviewed the literature and found that the inci- dence of wound metastasis was between 0% and 1.9% in the laparoscopic

Table 3
Randomized trials investigating reduction in hospital stay after laparoscopic colectomy

Author	Year	No. of patients	Length of stay	Significantly less than open
Stage [52]	1997	15	5	Yes
Schwenk [53]	1998	30	10.1	Yes
Milsom [40]	1998	54	5.2	no
Curet [42]	2000	18	5.2	Yes
Lacy [41]	2002	111	5.6	Yes
Weeks [47]	2002	168	7.1	Yes
Hasegawa [43]	2003	29	5	Yes
Nelson [48]	2004	345	5	Yes

group, and between 0.8% and 3.3% in the open surgery group [63]. It therefore appeared that the phenomenon of wound recurrence was not simply a laparoscopic problem. The major outcome of this was to prompt an increased interest in the biological aspects of the laparoscopic approach and its interface with the tumor, and the proposal of randomized trials. Multiple levels of evidence exist on the outcomes of laparoscopic colectomy. Many of the early trials give information on feasibility of approach, technical aspects, and personal experiences.

Only the results of powerful prospective randomized trials would help answer questions regarding oncological outcome of these patients undergoing laparoscopic resections. Many surgeons have continued to operate under the auspices of a trial on patients who have colorectal cancer; from this experience, many have produced useful prospective nonrandomized trials. Many of the nonrandomized prospective trials support the role of laparoscopic surgery for malignant disease, with a low recurrence rate and a lower incidence of port-site metastases than was reported in initial series. These also confirm the feasibility of the laparoscopic approach for colectomy, with comparable morbidity and mortality and oncological safety with open surgery. The only real negative comments are based on the significant increase in operative time caused by the laparoscopic approach.

The best evidence for the current status of laparoscopic surgery in oncology from the point of view of curative resection in colorectal cancer will come from large prospective randomized trials. The first randomized prospective trial comparing laparoscopic colectomy with open surgery was by Stage and coworkers in Denmark. In this small study, the feasibility and oncological safety of laparoscopic surgery were again demonstrated; however, conclusions were difficult because only 29 patients were included in the study analysis [52]. Larger studies, such as that by Lacy and coauthors in Europe, confirmed reports from nonrandomized trials and showed recurrence rates comparable with open surgery, and a low incidence of port-site metastases [64]. These trials acted as preludes to larger, multicenter prospective randomized trials. The three main trials are the COLOR trial, (COlon carcinoma Laparoscopic or Open Resection), a European multicenter randomized trial that began in 1997. In 27 hospitals in Sweden, the Netherlands, Germany, France, Italy, Spain, and the United Kingdom, 1200 patients will be included. The primary end point of the study is cancer-free survival after 3 years [65]. The US-based NCCTG trial will focus on disease-free survival, oncological resection, morbidity and mortality, and quality of life issues, as well as cost effectiveness [66]. The MRC-CLASICC trial, based in the United Kingdom, will examine adequacy of resection, and compare recurrence, morbidity and mortality rates, and disease-free survival [67]. The clinical outcomes of a surgical therapy study group compared 428 open colectomies and 435 laparoscopically assisted operations, and demonstrated quite clearly that recurrence and survival rates were similar in both groups. They found, however, a significant advantage for the laparoscopic group in

Table 4
Trials investigating recurrence and survival after laparoscopic colectomy

Author	Year	Study type	No. of patients	Recurrence %	Survival (year)	Survival %
Anderson [69]	2002	P	100	16.1	5	75.7
Scheidbach [70]	2002	P	206	11.6	5	80.9
Franklin [57]	1996	Cc	165	12.2	5	89.7
Schwandner [71]	1999	Cc	32	15.6	3	93
Hartley [72]	2001	Cc	21	5	3	71
Lacy [41]	2002	R	106	17	5	91
Nelson [48]	2004	R	345	0.5	4.4	77

Abbreviations: Cc, Case control; P, prospective; R, randomised.

analgesic requirement and length of stay [48]. Table 4 summarizes the results of many laparoscopic colectomy trials investigating overall recurrence rates and survival after surgery.

Initial reports from these randomized trials are positive and point to laparoscopic surgery having a positive role in them management of colorectal malignancies in the future [68].

Summary

The literature available on laparoscopic oncological surgery is varied; however, its role and status in modern surgical practice is becoming clearer. Its role in curative oncological resection still remains in the area of colo-rectal resection. Although it has been acceptable to continue laparoscopic surgery for colorectal disease, those who have subscribed have done so under the auspices of a trial many have continued their experiences with benign or palliative cases. Although we await the final reports from large randomized trials, it seems clear that with advancing learning curves and technology, the ease of operating has improved, leading to a decrease in operative times. Laparoscopic surgery also appears to be oncologically sound with regard to specimen resection, clearance, and lymph node harvest, and certainly comparable to open colectomy.

Although the true incidence of port-site metastases is difficult to ascertain, the initial fears of their occurrence in the early 1990s have not been realized by recently reports. It appears the phenomenon of port-site metastases was due to poor operative technique and learning curve issues, and that the technology of the time also played a role. Although the environment in which laparoscopic surgery is performed is different and has been shown at the physical and biological level to have effects on tumor cells, the role that this has in enhancement of tumor recurrence is still unclear. Reports from earlier nonrandomized series are demonstrating a wound recurrence rate not dissimilar to that of open surgery, and it is fully expected that results from randomized trials will support this.

Improved technique and experience with laparoscopic colectomy have demonstrated that morbidity and mortality levels are again similar to open operation; however, the distinct advantages of less pain, less wound infection, and improved cosmesis are beyond doubt. Once oncological safety has been demonstrated for the laparoscopic approach, the biggest questions to ask would be for curative resection. Does a laparoscopic approach support an earlier return to normal activity? Does it have positive effects on quality of life issues, and is it cost effective? Laparoscopic surgery for cancer has had to fight for surgical viability, and now has to demonstrate that it will deliver on its initial promise.

References

[1] Dobronte Z, Wittman T, Karacsony G. Rapid development of malignant metastases in the abdominal wall after laparoscopy. Endoscopy 1978;10:127–30.

[2] Sirimardena A, Samarji W. Cutaneous tumour seeding from a previously undiagnosed pancreatic carcinoma after laparoscopic cholecystectomy. Ann R Coll Surg Engl 1993;75: 199–200.

[3] Nduka CC, Monson JR, Menzies-Gow N, Darzi A. Abdominal wall metastases following laparoscopic surgery. Br J Surg 1994;81:648–52.

[4] Freeman RK, Wait MA. Port site metastasis after laparoscopic staging of esophageal carcinoma. Ann Thorac Surg 2001;71:1032–4.

[5] Cava A, Roman J, Gonzalez Quintela A, Martin F. Subcutaneous metastasis following laparoscopy in gastric adenocarcinoma. Eur J Surg Oncol 1990;16:63–7.

[6] Russi EG, Pergolizzi S, Mesiti M. Unusual relapse of hepatocellular carcinoma. Cancer 1992;70:1483–7.

[7] Elbahnasy AM, Hoenig DM, Shalav A. Laparoscopic staging of bladder tumour: concerns about port site metastases. J Endourol 1998;12:55–9.

[8] Wang PH, Yuan CC, Lin G. Risk factors contributing to early occurrence of port site metastases of laparoscopic surgery for malignancy. Gynecol Oncol 1999;72:38–44.

[9] Nauman RW, Spencer S. An umbilical metastasis after laparoscopy for squamous cell carcinoma of the cervix. Gynecol Oncol 1997;64:507–9.

[10] Kadar N. Port site recurrences following laparoscopic operations for gynaecological malignancies. Br J Obstet Gynaecol 1997;104:1308–13.

[11] Muntz HG, Goff BA, Madsen BL. Port site recurrence after laparoscopic surgery for endometrial carcinoma. Obstet Gynecol 1999;l3:807–9.

[12] Bacha EA, Barber W, Ratchford W. Port site metastases of adenocarcinoma of the fallopian tube after laparoscopically assisted vaginal hysterectomy and salpingo-oophorectomy. Surg Endosc 1996;10:1102–3.

[13] Morice P, Vaila J, Pautier P. Port site metastasis after laparoscopic surgery for gynaecologic cancer: a report of six cases. J Reprod Med 2000;45:837–40.

[14] Wexner SD, Cohen SM. Port site metastses after laparoscopic colorectal surgery for cure of malignancy. Br J Surg 1995;82:295–8.

[15] Whelan RL, Franklin M, Holubar SD. Post operative cell mediated immune response is better preserved after laparoscopic vs open colorectal resection in humans. Surg Endosc 2003;17:972–8.

[16] Carter JJ, Whelan. The immunologic consequences of laparoscopy in oncology. Surg Oncol Clin N Am 2001;10:655–77.

[17] Smith CD. Advanced laparoscopic procedures for the non-advanced laparoscopic surgeon. Int Surg 1994;79:259–65.

[18] Monson JR, Darzi A, Carey PD, Guillou PJ. Prospective evaluation of laparoscopic-assisted colectomy in an unselected group of patients. Lancett 1992;340:831–3.

[19] HALS Study Group. Hand assisted laparoscopic surgery vs standard laparoscopic surgery for colorectal disease: a prospective randomised trial. Surg Endosc 2000;14(10): 898–901.

[20] Bemelman WA, Ringers J, Meijer DW, et al. Laparoscopic assisted colectomy with dexterity pneumo sleeve. Dis Colon Rectum 1996;39(Suppl):S59–61.

[21] Ichiara T, Nagahata Y, Nomura H, et al. Laparoscopic lower anterior resection is equivalent to laparotomy for lower rectal cancer at the distal line of resection. Am J Surg 2000;43: 1164–7.

[22] Darzi A. Hand assisted laparoscopic colorectal surgery. Surg Endosc 2000;14:999–1004.

[23] Pietrabissa A, Moretto C, Carobbi A, et al. Hand assisted laparoscopic low anterior resection: initial experience with a new procedure. Surg Endosc 2002;16:431–5.

[24] Miura Y, Mitsuta H, Yoshihara T, et al. Gasless hand assisted laparoscopic laparoscopic surgery for colorectal cancer: an option for poor cardiopulmonary reserve. Dis Colon Rectum 2001;44:896–8.

[25] Nakajima K, Lee SW, Cocilovo C, et al. Hand assisted laparoscopic colorectal surgery using Gelport. Surg Endosc 2003;18:102–5.

[26] Jacobs M, Verdeja JC, Goldstein HS. Minimally invasive colon resection (laparoscopic colectomy). Surg Laparosc Endosc 1991;1:144–50.

[27] Falk PM, Beart RW, Wexner SD. Laparoscopic colectomy: a critical appraisal. Dis Colon Rectum 1993;36:28–34.

[28] Guillou PJ, Darzi A, Monson JR. Experience with laparoscopic colorectal surgery for malignant disease. Surg Oncol 1993;2:43–9.

[29] Milsom JW, Fazio VW. Concerns about laparoscopic colon cancer surgery. Dis Colon Rectum 1994;37:625–6.

[30] Stoker ME. Laparoscopic colon surgery for cancer: controversy, caution and common sense. Int Surg 1994;79:240–1.

[31] Wexner SD, Cohen SM, Johansen OB. Laparoscopic colorectal surgery: a prospective assessment and current perspective. Br J Surg 1993;80:1602–5.

[32] Darzi A, Lewis C, Menzies-Gow N, Monson JR. Laparoscopic abdomino-perineal excision of the rectum. Surg Endosc 1995;9:414–7.

[33] Fowler DL, White SA. Laparoscopic assisted sigmoid resection. Surg Laparosc Endosc Percutan Tech 1991;1:183–8.

[34] Schlinkert RT. Laparoscopic assisted right hemicolectomy. Dis Colon Rectum 1991;34: 1030–1.

[35] Phillips EH, Franklin M, Carroll BJ, et al. Laparoscopic colectomy. Ann Surg 1992;21: 703–7.

[36] Scoggin SD, Frazee RC, Snyder SK. Laparoscopic assisted bowel surgery. Dis Colon Rectum 1993;36:747–50.

[37] Peters WR, Bartels TL. Minimally invasive colectomy—are the potential benefits realized? Dis Colon Rectum 1993;36:751–6.

[38] Delgato S, Lacy AM, Garcia Valdecasas JC. Could age be an indication for laparoscopic surgery? Surg Endosc 2000;14:22–6.

[39] Schwenk W, Bohm B, Muller JM. Post operative pain and fatigue after laparoscopic or conventional colorectal resections. A prospective randomised trial. Surg Endosc 1998; 12:1131–6.

[40] Milsom JW, Bohm B, Hammerhoer KA, et al. A prospective randomised trial comparing laparoscopic versus conventional techniques in colorectal cancer surgery: a preliminary report. J Am Coll Surg 1998;187:46–7.

[41] Lacy AM, Garcia-Valdecasas J, Delgado S, et al. Laparoscopy assisted colectomy versus open colectomy for treatment of non-metastatic colon cancer: a randomised trial. Lancet 2002;359:2224–9.

[42] Curet MJ, Putrakul K, Pitcher DE, et al. Laparoscopically assisted colon resection for colon carcinoma: perioperative results and long term outcome. Surg Endosc 2000;14:1062–6.

[43] Hasegawa H, Kabeshima Y, Watanbe M, et al. Randomised controlled trial of laparoscopic versus open colectomy for advanced colorectal cancer. Surg Endosc 2003;17:631–40.

[44] Fritts LL, Orlando R, Thompson WR. Laparoscopic appendicectomy—safety and cost analysis. Arch Surg 1993;128:521–5.

[45] Bass EB, Pitt HA, Lillemoe KD. Cost effectiveness of laparoscopic cholecystectomy versus open cholecystectomy. Am J Surg 1993;165:466–71.

[46] Bokey EL, Moore JW, Chapuis PH. Morbidity and mortality following laparoscopic assisted right hemicolectomy for cancer. Dis Colon Rectum 1996;39:S24–8.

[47] Weeks JC, Nelson H, Gelber, et al. Short term quality of life outcomes following laparoscopic assisted colectomy versus open colectomy for colon cancer. A randomized trial. JAMA 2002;287:321–8.

[48] Nelson H, Sargent D, Fleshman J, et al. Clinical outcomes of surgical therapy study group of the laparoscopic colectomy trial. A comparison of laparoscopically assisted and open colectomy for colon cancer. N Engl J Med 2004;350:2050–9.

[49] Schideck THK, Schwandner O, Baca I. Laparoscopic surgery for the cure of colorectal cancer. Dis Colon Rectum 2000;43:1–8.

[50] Zhou ZG, Wang Z, Yu YY, et al. Laparoscopic total mesorectal excision of low rectal cancer with preservation of the anal sphincter report of 82 cases. World J Gastroenterol 2003;9: 1477–81.

[51] Tsang WWC, Chung CC, Li MKW. Prospective evaluation of laparoscopic total mesorectal excision with colonic J pouch reconstruction for mid and low rectal cancers. Br J Surg 2003; 90:867–71.

[52] Stage JG, Schulze S, Moller P. Prospective randomized study of laparoscopic versus open colonic resection for adenocarcinoma. Br J Surg 1997;84:1173–4.

[53] Schwenk W, Bohm B, Muller M. Postoperative pain and fatigue after laparoscopic or conventional colorectal resections. A prospective randomized trial. Surg Endosc 1998;12: 1131–6.

[54] Anderson CA, Kennedy FR, Potter M, et al. Results of laparoscopically assisted colon resection for carcinoma. The first 100 patients. Surg Endosc 2002;16:607–10.

[55] Moore JW, Bokey EL, Newland RC. Lymphovascular clearance in laparoscopically assisted right hemicolectomy is similar to open surgery. Aust N Z J Surg 1996;66:605–7.

[56] Lord SA, Larach SW, Ferrera A. Laparoscopic resections for colorectal carcinoma: a 3 year experience. Dis Colon Rectum 1996;39:148–54.

[57] Franklin ME, Rosenthal D, Abrego-Medina D. Prospective comparison of open versus laparoscopic resection of the colon and rectum for cancer. Dis Colon Rectum 1996;39:35–46.

[58] Decanini C, Milsom JW, Bohm B, Fazio VW. Laparoscopic oncologic abdomino-perineal resection. Dis Colon Rectum 1994;37:552–8.

[59] Abcarian H. Operative treatment of colorectal cancer. Cancer 1992;70(Suppl 5):1350–4.

[60] Corder AP, Karanjia ND, Williams JD, Heald RJ. Flush aortic tie versus selective preservation of the ascending left colic artery in low anterior resection for rectal carcinoma. Br J Surg 1992;79(7):680–2.

[61] Balli JE, Franklin ME, Almeida JA, Glass JL, Diaz JA, Reymond M. How to prevent port-site metastases in laparoscopic colorectal surgery. Surg Endosc 2000;14(11):1034–6.

[62] Wexner SD, Cohen SM. Port site metastases after laparoscopic colorectal surgery for cure of malignancy. Br J Surg 1995;82:295–8.

[63] Bonjer HJ, Lange JF, Jansen A. Abdominal metastasis following surgical removal of colorectal carcinoma. Ned Tijdschr Geneeskd 1997;27:1868–70.

[64] Lacy AM, Delgado S, Garcia-Valdecasas JC. Port site metastases and recurrence after laparoscopic colectomy. A randomized trial. Surg Endosc 1998;12:1039–42.

[65] Wittich PH, Kazemier G, Schouten WR. The colon cancer laparoscopic or open resection (COLOR trial). Ned Tijdsch Geneeskd 1997;141:1870–1.

[66] O'Connell MJ. Phase III randomized study of laparoscopic assited colectomy versus open colectomy for colon cancer. Cancernet. Available at: http://cancernet.nci.nih.gov/. Accessed December 2004.

[67] Guillou PJ. Phase III randomized study of conventional versus laparoscopic assited surgery for colorectal cancer. Cancernet. Available at: http://cancernet.nci.nih.gov/. Accessed December 2004.

[68] Hazebroek EJ. Color Study Group COLOR: a randomized clinical trial comparing laparoscopic and open resection for colon cancer. Surg Endosc 2002;16(6):949–53.

[69] Anderson CA, Kennedy FR, Potter M, et al. Results of laparoscopically assisted colon resection for carcinoma. The first 100 patients. Surg Endosc 2002;16:607–10.

[70] Schiedbach H, Schneider C, Konradt J, et al. Laparoscopic abdominoperineal resection and anterior resection with curative intent for carcinoma of the rectum. Surg Endosc 2002; 16:7–13.

[71] Schwandner O, Scheideck THK, Killaitis C, et al. A case control study comparing laparoscopic versus open surgery for rectosigmoidal and rectal cancer. Int J Colorectal Dis 1999;14:158–63.

[72] Hartley JE, Mehigan BJ, Quershi AE, et al. Total mesorectal excision: assessment of the laparoscopic approach. Dis Colon Rectum 2001;44:315–21.

ELSEVIER
SAUNDERS

SURGICAL
CLINICS OF
NORTH AMERICA

Surg Clin N Am 85 (2005) 61–73

Minimally invasive surgery for rectal cancer

W.W.C. Tsang, FRCSEd (Gen),
C.C. Chung, FRCSEd (Gen),
S.Y. Kwok, FRCSEd (Gen), M.K.W. Li, FRCS*

*Minimal Access Surgery Training Centre, Department of Surgery,
Pamela Youde Nethersole Eastern Hospital, 3 Lok Man Road, Chai Wan, Hong Kong*

Although enthusiasm for laparoscopic surgery in colon cancer sprouts with growing evidence of its oncological adequacy [1–8], most would not advocate its use in rectal cancer. Early reports on laparoscopic rectal cancer surgery were dominated by sphincter-ablating resection [9–15]. Technical hurdles as well as skepticism on oncological clearance had once confined sphincter preservation to carcinomas located at the rectosigmoid junction or in the upper rectum [8,16–20]. Progress in technology and skills, however, has finally led to the controversial extension of minimally invasive techniques to distal rectal cancer with sphincter preservation [21–33]. This article reviews the clinical outcomes of laparoscopic surgery for rectal cancer in the literature.

Radicality of resection

The oncologic basis of radical en-bloc resection for colorectal carcinoma lies in achieving a curative resection (RO) resection. In nonrandomized comparative studies, laparoscopic and open excision of rectal cancer were found to be equivalent in achieving distal and radial margins [9–12,18,24,28,33–35]; however, it is unclear whether sphincter preservation during laparoscopic total mesorectal excision (TME) puts the resection margins at greater risk. Small comparative studies found no difference in the distal [28,33] and radial margins [28] between laparoscopic and open sphincter-preserving TME. In four separate series, the reported distal

---

* Corresponding author.
E-mail address: mkwli@ha.org.hk (M.K.W. Li).

margin in laparoscopic sphincter-preserving TME for mid and low rectal cancer ranged from 3 to 4.3 cm, with microscopic involvement in 1% (range 0–2) of cases [27,29,30,33]. Bretagnol et al [29] reported a 7-mm radial margin with 10% microscopic involvement in 50 rectal tumors within 11 cm of anal verge. In two other series [27,30], all 131 patients who had carcinoma within 12 cm of the anal verge had tumor-free radial margins. The significance of microscopic margin involvement in some of these reports is hard to interpret, because they may reflect tumor characteristics rather than technical failure. Low rectal cancer, being surrounded by a thin meso-rectum, is associated with an increased rate of positive radial margin [36]. Long-term local recurrence rates for laparoscopic sphincter-preserving TME would be a more accurate and realistic measure of primary tumor clearance; however, there are limited recurrence data available [37,38].

The adequacy of radical resection can also be measured by the ability to achieve high-ligation, specimen characteristics, and lymph node yield. Scheidbach and colleagues [39] reported successful high ligation of the inferior mesenteric artery in 342 (90%) of 380 laparoscopic rectal cancer resections. Fleshmen and coauthors [9] showed equivalent rates of high ligation for laparoscopic and open abdominoperineal resection (APR). Rullier and collaborators [28] found intact fasica propria in 29 (91%) of 32 laparoscopic TME specimens, and demonstrated quality of excision comparable to open surgery. Except for one report [40], laparoscopic excision of rectal cancer was found to yield the same specimen length as open surgery in all comparative studies [10,24,33,35,41]. Finally, although lymph node harvest in the resected specimens varied considerably from 5.2 to 25 [9–12,18,24,25,27–29,32–35,39,40,42,43], this was found to be similar to that of open surgery in all [9–12,18,24,33–35] comparative studies but one [40].

The available evidence thus far suggests laparoscopic excision of rectal cancer is as radical as open surgery.

Safety and feasibility

There is now a wealth of evidence in the literature confirming the safety and feasibility of laparoscopic rectal cancer surgery. In the vast majority of reports, postoperative mortality rates following laparoscopic rectal cancer excision were low—the overall mortality rate in the literature is 1.3% (Table 1). Mortality rates were similar [9–12,24,28,34,40], and there was no increased overall morbidity [10–12,18,28,33,40,41,44] when compared with open surgery in most comparative studies (see Table 1). In Araujo et al's report [41], the only randomized study on laparoscopic versus open APR, there was zero mortality and no difference was observed between the two groups in terms of operative and postoperative complications.

One relevant safety issue is whether the laparoscopic approach alters the anastomotic leak rate of coloanal anastomosis. When diverting ileostomies are only selectively created, after laparoscopic sphincter-preserving TME

Table 1
Mortality and overall morbidity rates of laparoscopic rectal cancer surgery in the literature

Authors	Operation	No. of patients[a]		Mortality rate			Morbidity rate		
		Lap	Open	Lap	Open	p	Lap	Open	p
Darzi et al [12]	APR	12	16	8.3% (1)[a]	6.3% (1)	na	33.3%	56.3%	ns
Glattli et al [15]	APR	19	-	0%	-	-	42%	-	-
Ramos et al [10]	APR	20	18	0%	5.5% (1)	na	44%	66%	0.17
Iroatulum et al [11]	APR	8	7	0%	0%	na	25%	43%	na
Fleshman et al [9]	APR	42	152	0%	0%	na	69%	50%	na
Leung et al [50]	APR	25	34	0%	0%	ns	22	39	ns
Kockerling et al [43]	APR	116	-	1.7% (2)	-	-	34.4% (40)	-	-
Baker et al [34]	APR	28	61	3.6% (1)	3.3% (2)	na	36.9%	-	-
Scheidbach et al [39]	APR	149	-	2% (3)	-	-	38.1%	-	-
	AR	231	-	1.2% (3)	-	-		-	-
Schwander et al [18]	APR+AR	32	32	0%	3.1% (1)	na	31.3%	31.3%	na
Yamamoto et al [35]	APR+AR	70	-	0%	-	-	15%	-	-
Anthuber et al [40]	APR+AR	101	334	0%	1.5% (5)	0.175	10.9%	24.9%	0.003
Vorob et al [44]	AR	80	78	-	-	-	9.4%	25.6%	na
Weiser et al [21]	TME	21	-	-	-	-	14.3%	-	-
Watanabe et al [22]	TME	7	-	0%	-	-	14.3%	-	-
Hartley et al [24]	TME	42	22	0%	0%	na	26.2%	18.2%	na
Morino et al [27]	TME	100	-	2% (2)	-	-	36%	-	-
Ruiller et al [28][b]	TME	32	43	3.1% (1)	0%	0.427	21.9%	11.6%	0.340
Bretagnol et al [29][b]	TME	50	-	2% (1)	-	-	28%	-	-
Tsang et al [30]	TME	44	-	0%	-	-	34.1%	-	-
Zhou et al [31]	TME	82	-	0%	-	-	3.7%	-	-
Leroy et al [32]	TME	98	-	2% (2)	-	-	27%	-	-
Wu et al [33]	TME	18	18	-	-	-	5.6%	27.8%	<0.05
Total		1276[c]		1.3% (16)					

Abbreviations: APR, abdominoperineal resection; AR, anterior resection; Lap, laparoscopic; na, not available; ns, not significant; TME, total mesorectal excision.

[a] ( ), parentheses enclose number of patients.
[b] Studies on same group of patients.
[c] Total patient number in studies reporting on postoperative mortality after exclusion of patients duplicated in two studies noted by [a].

[24,27,32] the clinical leak rate was comparable to that of open TME and remained significant at 11% to 17% [45,46]. The authors practice routine protective ileostomy and have not experienced a single case of clinical leak, although 9% of our patients have had asymptomatic minor radiological leaks, as revealed by routine postoperative contrast enema [30]. Similarly, Bretagnol and coworkers [29] reported a 2% leakage rate with routine protective ileostomy. It is clear that anastomotic leaks are less frequent with proximal diversion [24,27,32], and when routinely employed following laparoscopic resection, comparable results can be achieved [47].

The feasibility of sphincter preservation following laparoscopic resection of distal rectal carcinoma relies not only on skills, but also on case selection. After exclusion of locally advanced tumors that invaded adjacent structures or the external anal sphincter, the authors achieved sphincter preservation in 44 cases of laparoscopic TME for cancers within 10 cm of anal verge, with a stapled anastomosis at 4 cm (range 2.5–5) [30]. Other single-surgeon series of laparoscopic sphincter-preserving TME have exercised similar case selection [27,29,33].

Feasibility of any laparoscopic procedure is reflected by its associated conversion rates. Conversion during laparoscopic rectal cancer excision varies greatly, from 0% to 33% [9–12,15,24,25,27,29–35,39–41,43,44]. Common reasons for conversion were intraoperative bleeding, bulky or locally advanced tumors, technical difficulties, and adhesions [9–11,24,25,27,29,31, 32,34,35,40]. The authors believe that timely conversion, wherever indicated, is of utmost importance in containing harm and should not be perceived as failure.

The long procedure time of certain laparoscopic rectal cancer operations is of interest. Laparoscopic APR quite consistently took an average of 3 to 4 hours among different reports [9–12,15,18,39,41,43]. The average operating time for laparoscopic sphincter-preserving TME was more variable, and ranged from 2 to 7 hours in different reports [21,22,27,28,30,31]. Although the difference might be due to variation in the surgical technique (stapled versus transanal intersphincteric dissection and hand-sewn anastomosis), case selection and patient habitus, the relatively long operating time supports the irrefutable fact that laparoscopic excision of low rectal cancer, though feasible, is technically demanding.

Postoperative outcomes

Although there is level one evidence showing that laparoscopic colectomy improves postoperative recovery [1–3,6–8,20,48,49], few studies on laparoscopic rectal cancer surgery have addressed this issue. Most are small and have produced conflicting results. Compared with open surgery, laparoscopic techniques may be associated with less operative blood loss and reduced perioperative transfusions [18,33,40], although there are data that indicate no difference [41]. There is also a marginal benefit in the length of hospital stay, with studies showing either similar [18,24,33,41] or shorter hospital stay [9–12,28,34,40]. The absolute reduction in the mean hospital stay was quite dramatic in the latter case, ranging from 4.5 to 7 days [9–12,28,34,40]. Evidence with regard to postoperative analgesic requirement is also unclear [10,18,24,44].

Of greater importance are the associated postoperative morbidities. With few exceptions [9,24], comparative studies showed either lower [11,33,40,44] or similar [10,12,18,28,41] overall morbidity rates when compared with open surgery (see Table 1). Because different investigators define morbidities differently, these data need to be interpreted with caution. It is more meaningful to examine and compare each specific morbidity separately. For instance, in Ramos et al's comparative study on APR [10], although the overall morbidity rates in the two groups were not significantly different (laparoscopic versus open = 44% versus 60%, $P = 0.17$; see Table 1), none of the patients in the laparoscopic group had abdominal wound complications, whereas six (33.3%) patients in the open group developed laparotomy wound infection ($P = 0.005$). The same findings was revealed by other investigators [12], though three other comparative studies on rectal cancer surgery reported a similar infection rate between the two techniques [18,24,33]. In a series by Leung and colleagues [50], although the overall morbidity rate in the two groups was no different, only two (8%) patients in the laparoscopic group (including converted cases) developed abdominal wound infection, whereas four (11.8%) patients in the open group suffered from either infection or major dehiscence in the laparotomy wound following APR. Additionally, none of the patients in the former group developed postoperative chest infection, whereas three patients (8.8%) in the latter had significant pneumonia. In the large series by Kockerling and coauthors on low rectal cancer [43], the incidences of abdominal wound disorders and chest infection were 5.1% and 4.3% respectively, converted cases being included. These figures are certainly noteworthy, and suggest that, as with laparoscopic colectomy, reduction in the size of the abdominal incision helps to decrease postoperative wound and pulmonary complications.

Port-site hernia as a complication specific to laparoscopic surgery had once raised concerns, especially among conservatives. In 16 studies [9–12,18, 21,22,24,25,27,29–33,39] that gave detailed accounts of postoperative complications, however, there were only three port-site hernias (0.3%) [9,21,30] among 1026 patients who had received laparoscopic rectal cancer surgery. Thus, port-site hernia is infrequent and should be avoidable with attention to port-site closure [51].

Postoperative bowel obstruction is yet another common morbidity following abdominal surgery. Although there is a suggestion from an animal study that adhesive obstruction might be less frequent after laparoscopic rectal cancer operations [52], there is little evidence for that in clinical settings. In several small comparative studies, the incidence of small bowel obstruction after laparoscopic rectal cancer excision was either the same as

[9] or just barely lower than [12,18,24] after open surgery. The small size of these studies and the lack of long-term follow-up means that any actual difference in the incidence of postoperative small bowel obstruction could have evaded detection.

Port-site metastasis

First reported in 1993 [53], port-site metastasis has stirred up much controversy against laparoscopic colectomy for malignancy. The incidences in recent series and randomized trials are much lower than those from initial reports [1,7,54,55]. Similarly, current evidence proves port-site metastasis to be a rare event in laparoscopic rectal cancer surgery. The overall incidence in the literature is 0.1% (Table 2), a figure comparable to that of wound recurrence in open surgery [56,57]. Thus, port-site metastasis is not an inherent detriment of laparoscopic surgery for rectal cancer.

Local recurrence and survival

Local recurrence is the single most important measure of success in rectal cancer surgery. The incidence varied dramatically, even among high-volume surgeons [58]. Surgeon factor, or more precisely the surgical technique, is a major determinant [58,59]. The technique of TME introduced by Heald in 1982 has set the standard for rectal cancer surgery, with a 10-year local recurrence rate of only 4% [37,60]. With such superb results from open surgery, local recurrence represents a major concern for laparoscopic

Table 2
Incidence of port-site metastasis after laparoscopic rectal cancer excision in the literature

Authors	Year	No. of patients	Port-site metastasis	
			No.	Percentage
Glattli et al [15]	1996	19	0	0
Ramos et al [10]	1997	20	0	0
Fleshman et al [9]	1999	42	0	0
Schwandner et al [18]	1999	32	0	0
Weiser et al [21]	2000	21	0	0
Hartley et al [24]	2001	42	0	0
Baker et al [34]	2002	28	0	0
Scheidbach et al [39]	2002	288	0	0
Yamamoto et al [25]	2002	70	0	0
Feliciotti F et al [35]	2003	48	0	0
Anthuber et al [40]	2003	101	0	0
Morino et al [27]	2003	70	1	1.4
Tsang et al [30]	2003	44	0	0
Zhou et al [31]	2003	82	0	0
Bretagnol et al [29]	2003	50	0	0
Leroy et al [32]	2004	98	0	0
Total		1055	1	0.1

surgery in rectal cancer. Table 3 shows the local recurrence rates of laparoscopic rectal cancer excision in different studies. These studies are often small, with short follow-up time, and a few [25,40] are made up of highly selected cases. The majority of the comparative studies found similar local recurrence rates for laparoscopic and open rectal cancer excision [9,10,24,34,5], and most were able to achieve a local recurrence rate below 10% (see Table 3). Of particular interest is the higher rate of local recurrence following laparoscopic APR when compared with sphincter-saving resections. Local recurrence rates after laparoscopic APR varied considerably, from 0% to 25% [9,10,18,34,39,41], whereas those of laparoscopic sphincter-saving TME were in the respectable range of 0% to 6% [24,27,29–32]. This phenomenon is analogous to that in open surgery [36,60,61]. Heald and coworkers had shown a much higher local recurrence rate after curative open APR (33%) than after anterior resection (1%) for

Table 3
Local recurrence rates after laparoscopic rectal cancer surgery in the literature

Authors	Year	Operation	No. of patients		FU (months)	Local recurrence rates		
			Lap	Open		Lap	Open	p
Ramos et al [10]	1997	APR	16	16	20*	6.3%	18.8%	0.28
Fleshman et al [9]	1999	APR	42	152	23.8*	19%	14%	ns
Baker et al [34]	2002	APR	28	61	35.6*	25%	32.8%	ns
Araujo et al [41]	2003	APR	13	13	47.2*	0%	15.4%	na
Schwandner et al [18]	1999	APR	13	13	40*	7.7%	0%	na
		AR	19	19	24.8*	0%	0%	na
Kockerling et al [43]	2000	APR	116	-	16**	7%	-	-
Barlehner et al [42]	2001	APR+AR	83	-	30**	1.2%	-	-
Scheidbach et al [39]	2002	APR	112	-	22.3*	9%	-	-
		+AR	176	-	25.9*	5.1%	-	-
Yamamoto et al [25]	2002	APR+AR	70	-	23**	2.9%	-	-
Feliciotti et al [35]	2003	APR+AR	48	33	43.8*	20.8%	18.2%	0.687
Anthuber et al [40]	2003	APR+AR	101	334	17**	2%	-	-
Hartley et al [24]	2001	TME	21	22	38**	5%	4.5%	1
Tsang et al [30]	2003	TME	44	-	15**	4.5%	-	-
Zhou et al [31]	2003	TME	82	-	1–24	2.4%	-	-
Morino et al [27]	2003	TME	70	-	45.7**	4.2%	-	-
Bretagnol et al [29]	2003	TME	50	-	18**	0%	-	-
Leroy et al [32]	2004	TME	98	-	36*	6%	-	-

Abbreviations: APR, abdominoperineal resection; AR, anterior resection; FU, follow-up; Lap, laparoscopic; na, not available; ns, not significant; TME, total mesorectal excision.
* Mean values.
** Median values.

tumors below 5 cm from the anal verge [61]. Likewise, The Norwegian Rectal Cancer Group reported a higher local recurrence rate for curative open APR (15%) than anterior resection (10%) in a cohort of 2136 cases of TME for distal two-third rectal cancer [36]. Although this might be due in part to the higher prevalence of T4 disease and positive radial margin in very low rectal cancer that had required sphincter ablation [36], conflicting evidence exists in the literature as to whether sphincter-ablating resection does alter the local recurrence rate in the treatment of low rectal cancer [36,61,62].

Long-term survival outcome presents the ultimate test for every cancer treatment modality. In the Norwegian study, the 5-year overall survival rates after curative APR and anterior resection were 55% and 68% respectively [36]. Long-term survival data of similar scale are currently unavailable for laparoscopic rectal cancer surgery. In fact, survival data on laparoscopic rectal cancer surgery are scanty in the literature, and follow-up time is short. In a multicenter study on 288 patients with a mean follow-up of 24.8 months, Scheidbach et al [39] reported 4-year overall survival rates of 86.6% and 71.7% after curative laparoscopic APR and anterior resection respectively. Morino and colleagues [27] reported 74% 5-year overall survival following curative laparoscopic TME, with a median follow-up of 46 months. With a mean follow-up of 3 years, Leroy and coworkers [32] reported a slightly lower 5-year figure of 65%. Several small comparative studies of laparoscopic versus open rectal cancer excision demonstrated no survival difference, but follow-up time was short in all these reports [9,18,24,34,35,44].

In short, although laparoscopic rectal cancer excision does not appear to confer any disadvantage in terms of early local disease recurrence and survival figures, such optimism needs to be substantiated by randomized controlled trials and long-term outcomes in the future.

Functional outcomes and cost

Genitourinary dysfunction after rectal cancer surgery is of paramount importance from the patient's perspective. Depending on the surgical procedures, adjuvant treatment, and the precise definition of dysfunction, the reported incidence of bladder dysfunction varied from 0% to 59% [63–68], and that of sexual dysfunction ranged from 0% to 75% [64–70]. Although sexual dysfunction is more commonly reported after sphincter-ablating surgery [68–70] and radiotherapy [64,69], there is evidence to suggest that the technique of TME apparently minimizes genitourinary dysfunction [65–67].

The few reports on genitourinary function after laparoscopic rectal cancer excision have yielded conflicting results. Rullier and collaborators [28] reported one (3.1%) long-term bladder dysfunction in 32 patients after laparoscopic TME and a 44% sexual dysfunction rate among male patients.

On the other hand, Watanabe et al [22] reported no genitourinary dysfunction in a small series of laparoscopic TME comprising only 7 patients. In the authors' series, although no patient suffered from long-term bladder dysfunction, 2 (9.5%) male patients complained of erectile dysfunction at follow-up visits [30]. Theoretically, with the magnified view and improved visualization of deep pelvic structures under the laparoscope [7,21,33], laparoscopic rectal cancer excision should yield functional outcomes at least comparable to, if not better than, open surgery. Nonetheless, data from Quah et al's study suggest that laparoscopic mesorectal excision might be associated with increased male sexual dysfunction [71]. In this study, however, the investigators used open technique to complete the distal rectal dissection, a technique which nerve damage is most likely with [72]. Currently, it remains unclear as to how laparoscopic approach affects genitourinary function after rectal cancer excision. This is not only because of the limited yet conflicting data, but also because different criteria and methods of measurement were employed in different reports. Clearly, genitourinary dysfunction must be addressed by future studies through objective and uniform assessments, such as urodyamnics and verified standard questionnaires [65,66].

No study has ever compared the cost of laparoscopic rectal cancer surgery with that of its open counterpart. Conflicting results from cost analysis studies of laparoscopic versus open colectomy [20,73–75] do not shed light on the subject. Because cost-effectiveness is of relevance in the overall assessment of the role of laparoscopic surgery in treating rectal cancer, such cost analysis studies are desperately needed in the future.

Summary

Current literature on laparoscopic rectal cancer surgery is limited and practically comprises only case series and nonrandomized, often small, comparative studies. The available evidence demonstrates its safety in experienced hands and an oncological clearance comparable to that of the open counterpart. Realistic case selection and timely conversion are crucial for success and avoiding harm. The design and size of the studies in the literature may have a part to play in the conflicting postoperative outcomes, which warrant clarification by large randomized trials. Amid the confusion, there is some suggestion of a marginal reduction in the operative blood loss and length of stay with the laparoscopic technique. Likewise, despite similar overall morbidity, there is level three evidence showing reduction in abdominal wound and pulmonary complications based on balance of probabilities. Data on genitourinary dysfunction after laparoscopic rectal cancer excision are currently very limited, and this needs to be addressed seriously in future studies. As far as oncological issues are concerned, port-site metastasis is rare and should not be a deterrent to laparoscopic surgery for rectal cancer. Laparoscopic surgery also does not seem to confer any disadvantage in early local disease recurrence and survival figures of rectal cancer. Having no adverse influence on postoperative and early oncological outcomes, laparoscopic rectal cancer surgery therefore deserves further evaluation, in the context of large randomized studies, to determine its functional and financial outcomes as well as long-term oncological outcomes.

References

[1] Lacy AM, Garcia-Valdecasas JC, Delgado S, Castells A, Taura P, Pique JM, et al. Laparoscopy-assisted colectomy versus open colectomy for treatment of non-metastatic colon cancer: a randomised trial. Lancet 2002;359(9325):2224–9.
[2] The Clinical Outcomes of Surgical Therapy Study Group. A comparison of laparoscopically assisted and open colectomy for colon cancer. N Engl J Med 2004;350(20):2050–9.
[3] Franklin ME Jr, Rosenthal D, Abrego-Medina D, Dorman JP, Glass JL, Norem R, et al. Prospective comparison of open vs. laparoscopic colon surgery for carcinoma. Five-year results. Dis Colon Rectum 1996;39(Suppl 10):S35–46.
[4] Hartley JE, Mehigan BJ, MacDonald AW, Lee PWR, Monson JRT. Patterns of recurrence and survival after laparoscopic and conventional resections for colorectal carcinoma. Ann Surg 2000;232(2):181–6.
[5] Patanker SK, Larach SW, Ferrara A, Williamson PR, Gallagher JT, DeJesus S, et al. Prospective comparison of laparoscopic vs. open resections for colorectal adenocarcinoma over a ten-year period. Dis Colon Rectum 2003;46(5):601–11.
[6] Champault GG, Barrat C, Raselli R, Elizalde A, Catheline JM. Laparoscopic versus open surgery for colorectal carcinoma: a prospective clinical trial involving 157 cases with a mean follow-up of 5 years. Surg Laparosc Endosc 2002;12(2):88–95.
[7] Chung CC, Tsang WWC, Kwok SY, Li MKW. Laparoscopy and its current role in the management of colorectal disease. Colorectal Dis 2003;5(6):528–43.
[8] Leung KL, Kwok SPY, Lau WY, Meng WCS, Lam TY, Kwong KH, et al. Laparoscopic-assisted resection of rectosigmoid carcinoma: immediate and medium-term results. Arch Surg 1997;132(7):761–4.
[9] Fleshman JW, Wexner SD, Anvari M, La Tulippe JF, Birnbaum EH, Kodner IJ, et al. Laparoscopic vs. open abdominoperineal resection for cancer. Dis Colon Rectum 1999; 42(7):930–9.
[10] Ramos JR, Petrosemolo RH, Valory EA, Polania FC, Pecanha R. Abdominoperineal resection: laparoscopic versus conventional. Surg Laparosc Endosc 1997;7(2):148–52.
[11] Iroatulam AJ, Agachan F, Alabaz O, Weiss EG, Nogueras JJ, Wexner SD. Laparoscopic abdominoperineal resection for anorectal cancer. Am Surg 1998;64(1):12–8.
[12] Darzi A, Lewis C, Menzies Gow N, Guillou PJ, Monson JR. Laparoscopic abdominoperineal excision of the rectum. Surg Endosc 1995;9(4):414–7.
[13] Chindasub S, Charntaracharmnong C, Nimitvanit C, Akkaranurukul P, Santitarmmanon B. Laparoscopic abdominoperineal resection. J Laparoendosc Surg 1994;4(1):17–21.
[14] Larach SW, Salomon MC, Williamson PR, Goldstein E. Laparoscopic assisted abdominoperineal resection. Surg Laparosc Endosc 1993;3(2):115–8.
[15] Glattli A, Birrer S, Buchmann P, Christen D, Frei E, Klaiber C, et al. Technick und resultate der laparoskopischen rektumexstirpation. (Technique and results of laparoscopic rectum resection.) Schweiz Med Wochenschr Suppl 1996;79:85S–8S. (in German)
[16] Goh YC, Eu KW, Seow-Choen F. Early postoperative results of a prospective series of laparoscopic vs. open anterior resections for rectosigmoid cancers. Dis Colon Rectum 1997; 40(7):776–80.

[17] Rhodes M, Rudd M, Nathanson L, Fielding G, Siu S, Hewett P, et al. Laparoscopic anterior resection: a consecutive series of 84 patients. Surg Laparosc Endosc 1996;6(3):213–7.

[18] Schwandner O, Schiedeck TH, Killaitis C, Bruch HP. A case-control-study comparing laparoscopic versus open surgery for rectosigmoidal and rectal cancer. Int J Colorectal Dis 1999;14(3):158–63.

[19] Scheidbach H, Schneider C, Baerlehner E, Konradt J, Koeckerling F. Laparoscopic anterior resection for rectal carcinoma. Results of a registry. Surg Oncol Clin N Am 2001;10(3): 599–609.

[20] Leung KL, Kwok SPY, Lam SCW, Lee JFY, Yiu RYC, Ng SSM, et al. Laparoscopic resection of rectosigmoid cancer: prospective randomized trial. Lancet 2004;363:1187–92.

[21] Weiser MR, Milsom JW. Laparoscopic total mesorectal excision with autonomic nerve preservation. Semin Surg Oncol 2000;19(4):396–403.

[22] Watanabe M, Teramoto T, Hasegawa H, Kitajima M. Laparoscopic ultralow anterior resection combined with per anum intersphincteric rectal dissection for lower rectal cancer. Dis Colon Rectum 2000;43(Suppl 10):S94–7.

[23] Chung CC, Ha JPY, Tsang WWC, Li MKW. Laparoscopic-assisted total mesorectal excision and colonic J pouch reconstruction in the treatment of rectal cancer. Surg Endosc 2001;15(10):1098–101.

[24] Hartley JE, Mehigan BJ, Qureshi AE, Duthie GS, Lee PWR, Monson JRT. Total mesorectal excision: assessment of the laparoscopic approach. Dis Colon Rectum 2001;44(3):315–21.

[25] Yamamoto S, Watanabe M, Hasegawa H, Kitajima M. Prospective evaluation of laparoscopic surgery for rectosigmoidal and rectal carcinoma. Dis Colon Rectum 2002; 45(12):1648–54.

[26] Pikarsky AJ, Rosenthal R, Weiss EG, Wexner SD. Laparoscopic total mesorectal excision. Surg Endosc 2002;16(4):558–62.

[27] Morino M, Parini U, Giraudo G, Salval M, Brachet Contul R, Garrone C. Laparoscopic total mesorectal excision: a consecutive series of 100 patients. Ann Surg 2003;237(3):335–42.

[28] Rullier E, Sa Cunha A, Couderc P, Rullier A, Gontier R, Saric J. Laparoscopic intersphincteric resection with coloplasty and coloanal anastomosis for mid and low rectal cancer. Br J Surg 2003;90(4):445–51.

[29] Bretagnol F, Rullier E, Couderc P, Rullier A, Saric J. Technical and oncological feasibility of laparoscopic total mesorectal excision with pouch coloanal anastomosis for rectal cancer. Colorectal Dis 2003;5(5):451–3.

[30] Tsang WWC, Chung CC, Li MKW. Prospective evaluation of laparoscopic total mesorectal excision with colonic J-pouch reconstruction for mid and low rectal cancers. Br J Surg 2003; 90(7):867–71.

[31] Zhou ZG, Wang Z, Yu YY, Shu Y, Cheng Z, Li L, et al. Laparoscopic total mesorectal excision of low rectal cancer with preservation of anal sphincter: a report of 82 cases. World J Gastroenterol 2003;9(7):1477–81.

[32] Leroy J, Jamali F, Forbes L, Smith M, Rubino F, Mutter D, et al. Laparoscopic total mesorectal excision (TME) for rectal cancer surgery: long term outcomes. Surg Endosc 2004; 18(2):281–9.

[33] Wu WX, Sun YM, Hua Y, Shen LZ. Laparoscopic versus conventional open resection of rectal carcinoma: a clinical comparative study. World J Gastroenterol 2004;10(8):1167–70.

[34] Baker RP, White EE, Titu L, Duthie GS, Lee PWR, Monson JRT. Does laparoscopic abdominoperineal resection of the rectum compromise long-term survival? Dis Colon Rectum 2002;45(11):1481–5.

[35] Feliciotti F, Guerrieri M, Paganini AM, De Sanctis A, Campagnacci R, Perretta S, et al. Long-term results of laparoscopic versus open resections for rectal cancer for 124 unselected patients. Surg Endosc 2003;17(10):1530–5.

[36] Wibe A, Syse A, Andersen E, Tretli S, Myrvold HE, Soreide O. Oncological outcomes after total mesorectal excision for cure for cancer of the lower rectum: anterior vs. abdominoperineal resection. Dis Colon Rectum 2004;47(1):48–58.

[37] Adam IJ, Mohamdee MO, Martin IG, Scott N, Finan PJ, Johnston D, et al. Role of circumferential margin involvement in local recurrence of rectal cancer. Lancet 1994; 344(8924):707–11.

[38] Heald RJ, Husband EM, Ryall RD. The mesorectum in rectal cancer surgery: the clue to pelvic recurrence? Br J Surg 1982;69(10):613–6.

[39] Scheidbach H, Schneider C, Konradt J, Barlehner E, Kohler L, Wittekind Ch, et al. Laparoscopic abdominoperineal resection and anterior resection with curative intent for carcinoma of the rectum. Surg Endosc 2002;16(1):7–13.

[40] Anthuber M, Fuerst A, Elser F, Berger R, Jauch KW. Outcome of laparoscopic surgery for rectal cancer in 101 patients. Dis Colon Rectum 2003;46(8):1047–53.

[41] Araujo SEA, da Silva e Sousa AH Jr, de Campos FGCM, Habr Gama A, Dumarco RB, Caravatto PP de P, et al. Conventional approach x laparoscopic abdominoperineal resection for rectal cancer treatment after neoadjuvant chemoradiation: results of a prospective randomized trial. Rev Hosp Clin Fac Med Sao Paulo 2003;58(3):133–40.

[42] Barlehner E, Decker T, Anders S, Heukrodt B. Laparoskopische chirurgie des rektumkarzinoms. Onkologische radikalitat und spatergebnisse. (Laparoscopic surgery of rectal carcinoma. Radical oncology and late results.) Zentralbl Chir 2001;126(4):302–6. (in German)

[43] Kockerling F, Scheidbach H, Schneider C, Barlehner E, Kohler L, Bruch HP, et al. Laparoscopic abdominoperineal resection: early postoperative results of a prospective study involving 116 patients. The Laparoscopic Colorectal Surgery Study Group. Dis Colon Rectum 2000;43(11):1503–11.

[44] Vorob ev GI, Shelygin Iu A, Frolov SA, Loshinin KV, Syshkov OI. Laparoskopicheskie operatsii u bol'nykh rakom priamoi kishki (sravnitel'nye rezul'taty laparoskopicheskikh otkrytykh perednikh rezektsii). (Laparoscopic surgery of rectal cancer (comparative results of laparoscopic and open abdominal resection).) Khirurgiia (Mosk) 2003;(3):36–42. (in Russian)

[45] Karanjia ND, Corder AP, Bearn P, Heald RJ. Leakage from stapled low anastomosis after total mesorectal excision for carcinoma of the rectum. Br J Surg 1994;81(8):1224–6.

[46] Carlsen E, Schlichting E, Guldvog I, Johnson E, Heald RJ. Effect of the introduction of total mesorectal excision for the treatment of rectal cancer. Br J Surg 1998;85(4):526–9.

[47] Karanjia ND, Corder AP, Holdsworth PJ, Heald RJ. Risk of peritonitis and fatal septicaemia and the need to defunction the low anastomosis. Br J Surg 1991;78(2): 196–8.

[48] Braga M, Vignali A, Gianotti L, Zuliani W, Radaelli G, Gruarin P, et al. Laparoscopic versus open colorectal surgery: a randomized trial on short-term outcome. Ann Surg 2002; 236(6):759–67.

[49] Chapman AE, Levitt MD, Hewett P, Woods R, Sheiner H, Maddern GJ. Laparoscopic-assisted resection of colorectal malignancies: a systematic review. Ann Surg 2001;234(5): 590–606.

[50] Leung KL, Kwok SPY, Lau WY, Meng WCS, Chung CC, Lai PBS, et al. Laparoscopic assisted abdominoperineal resection for low rectal cancer. Surg Endosc 2000;14: 67–70.

[51] Larach SW, Patankar SK, Ferrara A, Williamson PR, Perozo SE, Lord AS. Complications of laparoscopic colorectal surgery. Analysis and comparison of early vs. latter experience. Dis Colon Rectum 1997;40(5):592–6.

[52] Reissman P, Teoh TA, Skinner K, Burns JW, Wexner SD. Adhesion formation after laparoscopic anterior resection in a porcine model: a pilot study. Surg Laparosc Endosc 1996;6(2):136–9.

[53] Alexander RJ, Jaques BC, Mitchell KG. Laparoscopically assisted colectomy and wound recurrence. Lancet 1993;341(8839):249–50.

[54] Zmora O, Weiss EG. Trocar site recurrence in laparoscopic surgery for colorectal cancer. Myth or real concern? Surg Oncol Clin N Am 2001;10(3):625–38.

[55] Lacy AM, Delgado S, Garcia Valdecasas JC, Castells A, Pique JM, Grande L, et al. Port site metastasis and recurrence after laparoscopic colectomy. A randomized trial. Surg Endosc 1998;12(8):1039–42.

[56] Hughes ES, McDermott FT, Polglase AL, Johnson WR. Tumor recurrence in the abdominal wall scar tissue after large-bowel cancer surgery. Dis Colon Rectum 1983;26(9):571–2.

[57] Reilly WT, Nelson H, Schroeder G, Wieand HS, Bolton J, O'Connell MJ. Wound recurrence following conventional treatment of colorectal cancer: a rare but perhaps underestimated problem. Dis Colon Rectum 1996;39(2):200–7.

[58] Hermanek P. Impact of surgeon's technique on outcome after treatment of rectal carcinoma. Dis Colon Rectum 1999;42(5):559–62.

[59] Porter GA, Soskolne CL, Yakimets WW, Newman SC. Surgeon-related factors and outcome in rectal cancer. Ann Surg 1998;227(2):157–67.

[60] Heald RJ, Moran BJ, Ryall RD, Sexton R, MacFarlane JK. Rectal cancer: the Basingstoke experience of total mesorectal excision, 1978–1997. Arch Surg 1998;133(8):894–9.

[61] Heald RJ, Smedh RK, Kald A, Sexton R, Moran BJ. Abdominoperineal excision of the rectum—an endangered operation. Dis Colon Rectum 1997;40(7):747–51.

[62] Zaheer S, Pemberton JH, Farouk R, Dozois RR, Wolff BG, Ilstrup D. Surgical treatment of adenocarcinoma of the rectum. Ann Surg 1998;227(6):800–11.

[63] Fowler JW, Bremner DN, Moffat LE. The incidence and consequences of damage to the parasympathetic nerve supply to the bladder after abdominoperineal resection of the rectum for carcinoma. Br J Urol 1978;50(2):95–8.

[64] Bonnel C, Parc YR, Pocard M, Dehni N, Caplin S, Parc R, et al. Effects of preoperative radiotherapy for primary resectable rectal adenocarcinoma on male sexual and urinary function. Dis Colon Rectum 2002;45(7):934–9.

[65] Pocard M, Zinzindohoue F, Haab F, Caplin S, Parc R, Tiret E. A prospective study of sexual and urinary function before and after total mesorectal excision with autonomic nerve preservation for rectal cancer. Surgery 2002;131(4):368–72.

[66] Kim NK, Aahn TW, Park JK, Lee KY, Lee WH, Sohn SK, et al. Assessment of sexual and voiding function after total mesorectal excision with pelvic autonomic nerve preservation in males with rectal cancer. Dis Colon Rectum 2002;45(9):1178–85.

[67] Havenga K, Enker WE, McDermott K, Cohen AM, Minsky BD, Guillem J. Male and female sexual and urinary function after total mesorectal excision with autonomic nerve preservation for carcinoma of the rectum. J Am Coll Surg 1996;182(6):495–502.

[68] Cosimelli M, Mannella E, Giannarelli D, Casaldi V, Wappner G, Cavaliere F, et al. Nerve-sparing surgery in 302 resectable rectosigmoid cancer patients: genitourinary morbidity and 10-year survival. Dis Colon Rectum 1994;37(Suppl 2):S42–6.

[69] Chorost MI, Weber TK, Lee RJ, Rodriguez Bigas MA, Petrelli NJ. Sexual dysfunction, informed consent and multimodality therapy for rectal cancer. Am J Surg 2000;179(4):271–4.

[70] Keating JP. Sexual function after rectal excision. Aust N Z J Surg 2004;74(4):248–59.

[71] Quah HM, Jayne DG, Eu KW, Seow-Choen F. Bladder and sexual dysfunction following laparoscopically assisted and conventional open mesorectal resection for cancer. Br J Surg 2002;89(12):1551–6.

[72] Rubino F, Leroy J, Marescaux J. Bladder and sexual dysfunction following laparoscopically assisted and conventional open mesorectal resection for cancer (Br J Surg 2002;89:1551–6). Br J Surg 2003;90(4):486.

[73] Philipson BM, Bokey EL, Moore JW, Chapuis PH, Bagge E. Cost of open versus laparosocopically assisted right hemicolectomy for cancer. World J Surg 1997;21(2):214–7.

[74] Falk PM, Beart RW Jr, Wexner SD, Thorson AG, Jagleman DG, Lavery IC, et al. Laparoscopic colectomy: a critical appraisal. Dis Colon Rectum 1993;36(1):28–34.

[75] Delaney CP, Kiran RP, Senagore AJ, Brady K, Fazio VW. Case-matched comparison of clinical and financial outcome after laparoscopic or open colorectal surgery. Ann Surg 2003;238(1):67–72.

ELSEVIER
SAUNDERS

Surg Clin N Am 85 (2005) 75–90

SURGICAL
CLINICS OF
NORTH AMERICA

Laparoscopic surgery of the spleen

Selman Uranues, MD, FACS[a],*, Orhan Alimoglu, MD[b]

[a]*Department of Surgery, Medical University of Graz, Auenbruggerplatz 29,
8036 Graz, Austria*
[b]*Department of Surgery, Vakif Teaching Hospital, Istanbul, Turkey*

Not very long ago, it was assumed that the spleen, which Galen had called an "organum plenum mysterii," could be removed without reservations. In antiquity, there had been all sorts of beliefs about the function and significance of the spleen. The spleen was regarded by Diogenes, Hippocrates, Plato, and Galen as an organ for the conservation of eucrasia and emotional equilibrium, as a receptacle for black bile, and as an equally important counterpart to the liver [1]. Based on Galen's description, the spleen was long assumed to be a part of the digestive tract, with a connecting duct to the liver. It was not until 1686 that Malpighi demonstrated the follicular and trabecular structure of the spleen and that it had its own arterial and venous circulation. The first planned, successful splenectomy was performed in the 16th century. In 1549, Zaccarello of Palo, a famous surgeon, completely removed an enlarged spleen from a young woman. Later writers have inferred from the description that a large ovarian cyst was actually removed [2]. The first successful splenectomy following primary splenic rupture was reported in 1893 by Riegner [3]. In 1896, Lamarchia successfully conserved a spleen by suturing the capsule after a delayed rupture. The literature from the seventeenth, eighteenth and nineteenth centuries includes further isolated case reports on partial resections and splenectomies for the most varied indications. The great surgeons of this period, such as Spencer Wells, Billroth, Volkman, Martin, Pean, Czerny, and Trendelenburg, reported successful splenectomies [2].

Before the turn of the 19th century, Ehrlich and Vulpius first suggested that the spleen could play a role in resistance [1]. In 1919, Morris and Bullock showed the influence of the spleen on resistance to infection in animal experiments. O'Donnel reported the first human case of fatal postsplenectomy sepsis in 1929. In 1952, King and Shumacker suggested the relationship of

---

* Corresponding author.
E-mail address: selman.uranues@meduni-graz.at (S. Uranues).

0039-6109/05/$ - see front matter © 2005 Elsevier Inc. All rights reserved.
doi:10.1016/j.suc.2004.09.003
surgical.theclinics.com

increased susceptibility to infection in splenectomized patients to the splenectomy [4]. Others soon confirmed that severe infection and death in children due to fulminating sepsis occurred after splenectomy [5].

In a retrospective analysis of 2796 splenectomized patients, Singer [6] found 119 (4.25%) cases of septic infections. Seventy-one patients (2.52% of the total patients and 60% of the sepsis cases) died of sepsis. Sepsis as cause of death is 200 times more common in splenectomized patients than in the general population, in which Singer reports an incidence of sepsis mortality of 0.01% [6]. The respective rates are 0.58% in post-traumatic splenectomy patients, 0.85% after incidental splenectomy, and even higher following splenectomy for hematological reasons (thalassemia 11%, hemolytic anemia 2.9%, portal hypertension 5.9%). The most common pathogens are *Streptococcus pneumoniae* and other species, *Neisseria meningitidis*, *Hemophilus influenzae*, *Escherichia coli*, and *Staphylococcus* spp.

The real revolution in surgical handling was introduced by the pioneering work of the Brazilian surgeon Marcel Campos Christo and Leon Morgenstern in the early 1960s and 1970s. Christo first reported experimental segmental splenectomy in animals. Then he applied these techniques to eight patients who had splenic injuries [7]. In 1966, Morgenstern reported subtotal splenectomies for hematological disease [8]. These publications on partial splenic conservation in trauma and massive splenomegaly attracted the attention of not only pediatric but also general surgeons. In the 1980s and 1990s, staplers for partial resection of the spleen were introduced [9].

After the dawn of the laparoscopic era, it was not very long until Delaitre [10] reported the first laparoscopic splenectomy. Shortly after the first publications of laparoscopic splenectomies, experimental and then clinical laparoscopic partial resections of the spleen were reported [11]. Today, nearly 20 years after the laparoscopy revolution in surgery, laparoscopic splenectomy is standard procedure for patients who have a hematological diagnosis and a normal-sized or moderately enlarged spleen. Open procedure is used only for excessively enlarged spleens.

Operations on the spleen can be divided into two groups: laparoscopic total splenectomy and laparoscopic partial splenectomy. Both are discussed in the following, with particular attention to laparoscopic partial resection.

Selection criteria and indications

Most suitable for laparoscopic technique is a spleen that is either not enlarged at all, or that has a sonographically measured cranio-caudal long axis of not more than 20 cm. Larger spleens can be removed in a laparoscopically assisted operation with a laparoscopy hand port. Spleens with a long axis of more than 30 cm demand unfavorable trocar placement, and removal of the specimen can require such a long incision that it does not make sense to attempt a laparoscopic procedure.

The indications for laparoscopic splenectomy are generally the same as those for open technique (Table 1). Indications for splenectomy aim to achieve one of three therapeutic goals:

1. Prevention of elimination of corpuscular elements of the blood in the pulpa of the spleen in any of the three types of congenital red-cell disorders that are associated with decreased erythrocyte deformability and cause anemias: disorders of the erythrocyte membranes, hemoglobinopathies, and erythrocyte enzyme deficiencies
2. Treatment of splenomegaly and hypersplenism
3. Staging of disease; eg, Hodgkin's disease

The most common indications for laparoscopic hemisplenectomy are benign primary lesions such as cysts and hamartomas (Table 2). When they are larger than 2 to 3 cm, they usually cause complaints of varying severity. Depending on the size of the lesion, the symptoms can range from diffuse upper abdominal pain to respiratory distress when lying down. Larger cysts can often displace or compress neighboring organs. Cysts larger than 5 cm are much more likely to rupture with even minor trauma. In two of the authors' cases, bleeding within the cyst caused symptoms resembling those of a heart attack; the patients were admitted to a medical service for evaluation of the cardiac situation.

Preoperative preparation

Preoperative preparation for a partial splenectomy is the same as for a total splenectomy. Because the possibility can never be excluded that what

Table 1
General indications for splenectomy

Hemolytic anemias	Purpuras	Secondary hypersplenism	Primary hematologic diseases	Other disorders
Hereditary spherocytosis	Idiopathic thrombocytopenic purpura (ITP)	Cirrhosis	Lymphoma	Pancytopenia in Felty's syndrome
Elliptocytosis		Cystic fibrosis	Chronic lymphocytic leukemia	Sarcoidosis
Enzyme-deficient hemolytic anemia	Thrombotic thrombocytopenic purpura (TTP)	Myelo- and lympho proliferative disorders	Myeloid metaplasia	Gaucher's disease
Thalassemia			Myelo- and lympho proliferative disorders	Abscesses
Sickle cell disease				Infarcts
Idiopathic autoimmune haemolytic anemia				Splenic artery aneurysms
				Cysts, Tumors

Table 2
Indications for partial splenic resection

Diagnostic	Therapeutic	Due to injury
Splenomegaly of unknown origin	Splenic cysts (except parasitic) Benign tumors (hamartoma, fibroma, pulpoma) Metastases (gynaecological) Infarcts Intrasplenic pancreatic cysts	Nontraumatic accidental lacerations

was intended to be a partial resection may end in a total splenectomy, candidates for partial resection should also be immunized against pneumococcus at least 1 week, but preferably somewhat longer, before surgery, and informed accordingly. In case of splenectomy, if the immunization was not administered before surgery, it can be given 1 or 2 weeks thereafter. The patient should be free of infections upon immunization; this applies to children as well. Long-term antibiotic prophylaxis has not as yet been proven to be advantageous in preventing infections. Nonetheless, even years after a splenectomy, antibiotics should be prescribed generously at the very first sign of an infection.

Positioning of the patient and of the trocars

In laparoscopic splenic surgery, the position of the patient is at least as important as the choice of trocar sites. The patient lies in a semilateral position on the right side with the left arm fixed over the head in a splint. This permits a better approach to the spleen via the left thoracic aperture. The lateral axis of the body from shoulder blade to shoulder blade is at an angle of 45° to 60° to the surface of the operating table (Fig. 1). The patient's body is somewhat overextended. In this position, the spleen hangs from its dorsolateral fixation and the other organs shift caudally, and the approach to the splenic hilus is easier. By turning the operating table, the patient can be brought into a supine position to facilitate the search for accessory spleens.

The use of three to four trocars is appropriate in most cases (Fig. 2). The trocar positions should be chosen carefully on the basis of the size of the spleen. The first trocar is inserted in the umbilical region, as is usual in open technique, and serves as the camera port. It is standard practice to use a 30° optic. A 5 to 12 mm trocar is inserted on the left medioclavicular line, either cranially or caudally from the level of the umbilicus, depending on the size of the spleen. It serves initially as the working trocar, and the endostapler is also inserted through it to sever the splenic vessels. The third trocar, with a diameter of 5 to 12 mm, is placed in the epigastric region, paramedially and on the left or right, depending on the size of the spleen; it is the second working trocar and is used to introduce a grasper, a suction device, or an

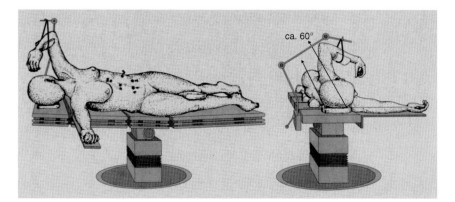

Fig. 1. Positioning of the patient.

endostapler. For the transsection of the splenic parenchyma, the endostapler is inserted from the medial direction. These three trocars generally suffice. In exceptional cases, a fourth 5-mm trocar for a retractor can be inserted subcostally in the left side in the anterior axillary line or subxiphoidally.

Operative procedure

First step: mobilization

For the partial resection, the operation begins with mobilization of the spleen. Unlike an open partial resection, with laparoscopic technique only that part of the spleen that is to be resected is mobilized. If the lower half of the spleen is to be removed, the omental connections including the branches of the gastroepiploic artery are first severed, most suitably with ultrasonic scissors or the Ligasure instrument (Valleylab, Boulder, Colorado).

If the upper half is to be removed (Fig. 3), mobilization begins with the visceral surface at the planned resection line above the entry of the main

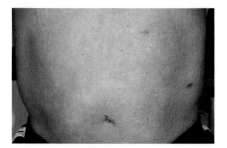

Fig. 2. Scars after laparoscopic partial resection.

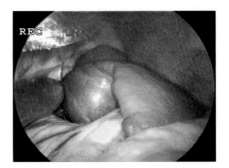

Fig. 3. Upper pole hamartoma in a 13-year-old girl.

vessels. After the omental connections and the short gastric vessels have been severed, the upper pole artery is presented (Fig. 4).

Second step: vascular dissection

The vascular dissection depends on the extent of resection. The authors find that there are three possibilities:

1. The lesion is located in the supply area of the upper or lower polar vessel. In this case, it suffices to dissect the vessel with the Ligasure instrument (Fig. 5) or clips.
2. The lesion extends beyond the supply area of the respective polar vessel into that of the main vessel, but is still peripheral and does not touch the hilus. In this case, after ligature of the respective polar vessel, the lesion is dissected out of the parenchyma. The parenchymal surface is closed with a running suture.
3. The part of the spleen that is to be removed begins at one pole and extends over the middle segment into the supply area of the other polar vessel. In these cases, a subtotal resection is indicated, and this will only be possible if the vessel that is to be preserved branches off early. The

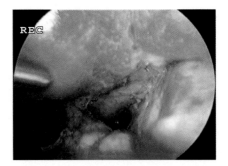

Fig. 4. Dissection of the upper pole artery (same patient as in Fig. 3).

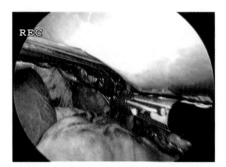

Fig. 5. Upper pole artery severed with Ligasure (same patient as in Fig. 3).

main vessels, the splenic artery and vein, and the respective polar vessel are severed with the endostapler. In this case, the endostapler is inserted from caudal through a 12 mm trocar in the medioclavicular line.

Third step: parenchymal resection

With few exceptions, the parenchyma can be transected with an endostapler using a blue 60 mm parenchymal cartridge (Fig. 6A, B). The parenchyma is compressed with a long, atraumatic grasper on the planned transsection line that the previous vascular dissection has rendered clearly visible. Compression is applied slowly and stepwise to avoid injury to the capsule. Only when the parenchyma is sufficiently compressed is the endostapler introduced through the epigastric 12 mm trocar and the resection performed, usually in two steps (Fig. 7).

Fourth step: sealing and tamponading the transected edge and removal of the specimen

In both splenectomies and partial resections, the use of hemostyptic substances such as collagen fleece or fibrin adhesive has proven to be valuable when there is a pronounced tendency to bleed, as for example with hepatic cirrhosis, coagulopathies, and thrombocytopenia. The authors routinely use a suitable laparoscopic device to spray the entire wound area with autologous fibrin sealant (Vivostat, Vivolution A/S, Denmark) and tamponade the stumps of the blood vessels and the cut edge of the spleen with collagen fleece (Lysostypt, Braun AG, Germany). Both the fibrin adhesive and the collagen fleece quickly help the spleen adhere to its surroundings and thus reduce the likelihood of torsion or venous buckling.

Only in exceptional cases is it necessary to drain the splenic fossa; the drain is removed on the second postoperative day at the latest.

The last step is the removal of the specimen. The spleen should always be placed in a waterproof endobag. Enlarged spleens will require larger pouches, which can be introduced without a trocar through the enlarged umbilical

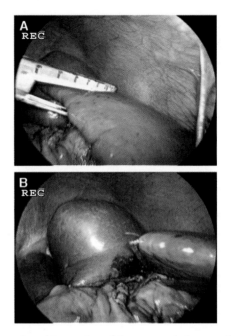

Fig. 6. (*A,B*) Parenchymal transection of the upper pole (same patient as in Fig. 3).

trocar incision. Usually the specimen will be fragmented and so removed through a smaller incision. It is important to avoid accidental splenosis through spreading of particles of the splenic parenchyma in the abdomen.

Postoperative management

A nasogastric tube should be left in place until the patient has completely regained consciousness. Oral feeding can begin at the same day. One-shot perioperative antibiotic prophylaxis with broadband antibiotics is highly

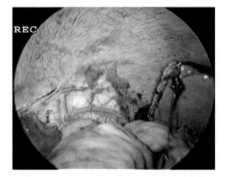

Fig. 7. Stapled resection margin of the remaining lower half of the spleen (same patient as in Fig. 3).

appropriate. Depending on the circulatory situation, patients can be mobilized on the day of surgery. Thrombosis prophylaxis should be routine, depending on the coagulation status. Physical activity is not limited after either a laparoscopic splenectomy or a laparoscopic partial splenectomy.

Patients

From 1994 to 2003, there were 143 elective splenectomies and 43 nontraumatic partial resections (Table 3).

Open splenectomy

Eighty-two of 143 operations were performed with open technique. There were four splenic abscesses, and 2 patients had multiple splenic infarcts and were in such poor condition that a laparoscopic procedure was not an option. The remaining 76 patients had hematological diseases, with pronounced splenomegaly and spleens weighing 900 to 4240 g. On the average, two units of blood were required in open splenectomy (Table 4). Four patients (4.8%) died in the postoperative phase: 3 of cardiopulmonary failure and 1 of acute thrombosis of the portal vein. Within 2 years after open splenectomy, 52% of patients developed an incisional hernia of varying size in the area of the median laparotomy scar.

Laparoscopic splenectomy

In the same period, 61 patients underwent laparoscopic splenectomy. The criteria for laparoscopy were suitable physical condition as well as the sonographically measured long axis of the spleen, which was not to exceed 20 cm. With these selection criteria, all of the extirpated spleens weighed less than 800 g. There were 44 patients who had idiopathic thrombocytopenic purpura (ITP) and thrombotic thrombocytopenic purpura (TTP), 10 who

Table 3
Patients with splenic procedures (1994–2003)

Procedure	No. of patients	Spleen weight (g)	Operation time (min.)	Postoperative complications (%)	Mortality
Open splenectomy	82	900–4240	94	28.9	4.8
Laparoscopic splenectomy	61	up to 800	108	6.4	0
Open partial splenectomy	12	Not applicable	117	4.9	0
Laparoscopic partial splenectomy	31	Not applicable	110	1.6	0

had chronic anemia, 4 who had malignant lymphoma, and 1 who had a solitary splenic metastasis after ovarian carcinoma. Conversion to open technique was required twice (3.2%) due to venous hilar hemorrhage; once in the case of a lymphoma and once in an ITP patient. The lowest thrombocyte count among the nonconverted purpura patients was 9000. There were no deaths in this group.

Open partial resection

Twelve patients underwent nontraumatic open hemisplenectomy (Table 5). With the exception of 1 patient who had a solitary metastasis, all of them had surgery before the year 2000. From 1999 onwards, partial splenectomies were performed with laparoscopic technique more and more often, and in the last 3 years, from 2001 onward, exclusively so. The patients who had open partial resection included three cases with subtotal splenectomies in two children aged 13 and 15, and a 19-year-old woman who had massive splenomegaly in the context of cystic fibrosis and cirrhosis of the liver. The extirpated splenic specimens weighed 1900 to 3000 g. The young woman's remaining spleen had to be removed 24 hours after surgery due to thrombotic occlusion of the remaining upper polar vessel. Seven further patients had congenital cysts. Two patients underwent partial resections due to solitary gynecological metastases. There were no deaths. The children who had cystic fibrosis required blood transfusions. The young woman whose residual spleen was removed 24 hours after surgery required three units of packed erythrocytes, whereas the two children each received two. Two patients (3.2%) developed incisional hernias.

Laparoscopic partial resection

A total of 31 patients underwent a laparoscopic partial splenectomy, whereby the lower pole was involved in 10, and in 16 the upper pole was resected (see Table 5). Three patients had a subtotal resection; 2 of them for extensive cysts and 1, a 14-year-old girl, for reduction of the size of the organ in the context of spherocytosis. One patient had to be converted to open technique; there were no mortalities.

Splenic cysts were the indication for surgery in 19 patients aged 14 to 62, 4 of them for cyst recurrences. All of the latter had undergone a deroofing procedure. A 13-year-old girl had had two laparoscopic operations and an 18-year-old woman had had open surgery. The cysts always recurred within a few months and were abundantly symptomatic.

There were five operations for hamartomas: the youngest patient was 13 years old and the oldest, 72. Two patients had a partial splenectomy for a splenic metastasis of an ovarian carcinoma and of a schwannoma.

Only two patients required blood transfusions. The 14-year-old spherocytosis patient received two units and the 72-year-old man who had

Table 4
Splenectomy for hematologic disease

Author	No. of patients Malignant/benign		Spleen weight Malignant/benign		Operation method Laparoscopic/open		Operation time (min.) Laparoscopic/open		Postoperative complications (%) Malignant/benign		Mortality (%) Malignant/benign		Conversion (%) Malignant/benign	
Horowitz 1996 [27]	135	0	120–3500		open				52		9			
Schlachta 1999 [28]	11	47			laparoscopic		239	180	18	11	9	0	21	6
Donini 1999 [29]	106		733	732	44	56	130	133	LS 7	OS 23	0	0		
Park 1999 [30]	210		264	284	147	63	145	77	LS 10.2	OS 24.9			2.7	
Authors' series	143		LS <800	OS 900–4240	61	82	108	94	LS 4	OS 28.9	0	4.8	3.2	

Abbreviations: LS, laparoscopic splenectomy; OS, open splenectomy.

Table 5
Partial splenectomy

Operation	No. of patients	Type of resection	Operation time (min.)	Blood transfusion	Postop. complications (%)	Mortality	Conversion
Open	12	Upper pole: 3 Lower pole: 5 Subtotal: 4	117	3 patients	4.9	0	1 reoperation for splenectomy
Laparoscopic	31	Upper pole: 16 Lower pole: 10 Subtotal: 3	110	2 patients	1.6	0	2

a hamartoma of 7 cm diameter received three units of packed erythrocytes. There were no incisional hernias.

Discussion

The past 2 decades have seen major changes in the treatment of splenic disorders. These changes evolved based on the concept that splenectomy renders patients at lifelong risk for increased susceptibility to infections. The most serious of these infections is the overwhelming postsplenectomy infection, which occurs in about 0.5% of trauma patients, and in up to 20% of patients who have hematologic disorders. When postsplenectomy sepsis occurs, mortality is very high—up to 80%. This risk is greatest in the first 2 years of asplenism and persists throughout life. This danger is also present when an adult undergoes a traumatic splenectomy. Sepsis can also occur even after splenic preservation, sometimes many years thereafter [12], when the spleen is not supplied by its main blood vessel. This has also been seen to be the case with post-traumatic autologous spleen transplant, and in asplenic patients with accessory spleens or splenosis. In these cases as well, the available splenic parenchyma does not offer sufficient protection against infections [13–17].

The authors believe that the high rate of blood flow through the organ is the reason for the spleen's great immunological competence. The spleen weighs some 120 g and 10 L of blood per hour flow through the organ. It contains more lymphatic tissue than all of the lymph nodes in the human body taken together. It is, however, directly connected to the circulatory system and has no afferent lymph vessels.

For these reasons, a trend away from splenectomy and toward splenic conservation has emerged. In trauma patients, spleen-preserving operations remain within the domain of open surgery [18,19], but benign splenic tumors can be resected with spleen-conserving laparoscopic technique. An important point that seems to the authors to be very different from open technique and that should be borne in mind is that with laparoscopic partial resection, only that part of the spleen should be mobilized that is to be removed. This serves to prevent torsion or buckling of the hilar vessels [20].

A second point that should be emphasized is that deroofing of congenital cysts is not a satisfactory treatment, and in the authors' experience it almost always leads to recurrences [9,21–23]. We operated on four patients who had recurring cysts. All of them had had previous primary open or laparoscopic deroofing procedures, and a 14-year-old girl had in fact undergone two previous laparoscopic operations within 1 year. These four patients have remained free of cysts and complaints following laparoscopic hemi-splenectomy of the cyst-bearing portion of the spleen.

We find that precise preoperative imaging of the hilar vessels is a prerequisite for a successful and unbloody partial resection of the spleen; this can be achieved with contrast computer tomography or magnetic resonance angiography. The surgeon can see the extent of the lesion and the vascular supply in this area, and can determine the extent of the resection. Postoperative immunological competence depends on adequate perfusion by the splenic artery or a large upper or lower polar artery. If the splenic artery must be severed, the severance should be pre-hilar, after the respective polar vessel has branched off. We have so treated our patients, and none of them has developed operation-specific complications. The two converted patients in the laparoscopic splenectomy group underwent surgery with hemoclips before the advent of modern coagulation technique with ultrasonic scissors and the Ligasure instrument. In both cases, hemorrhage from the splenic vein forced us to convert. The techniques of ultrasonic coagulation and the Ligasure instrument have contributed importantly to the fact that today, total and partial splenectomy can be performed safely and quickly with laparoscopic technique [24].

A patient undergoing laparoscopic partial resection had to be converted because of an excessively large congenital cyst, with a partially sclerotic wall that could not be cut with laparoscopic instruments. The procedure was completed as an open partial splenectomy.

With benign lesions, organ preservation should always be attempted, but patients who have malignant hematological diseases usually require splenectomy. Laparoscopic technique offers the usual advantages with splenectomy as with other procedures. This is especially striking with scar hernias, where we have found a significant difference between open and laparoscopic technique in our patient collective, with an incidence of 52% after open splenectomy after 2 years versus 3.2% for laparoscopic procedures [25].

Independent of the defect in the immune-defense system against encapsulated cocci due to splenectomy, in laparoscopic surgery the postoperative complication rate is significantly lower than for open splenectomy [26–30].

Laparoscopic splenectomy is already standard for ITP and TTP [31–34]. Both the authors' own experience and the cited literature show that the duration of surgery with normal to moderately enlarged spleens is about the same for laparoscopic and open procedures (see Table 5). As the number of laparoscopic operations performed increases, the length of surgery decreases until it is less than that for open technique. Laparoscopic technique is, however, limited by the size of the spleen. In cases with massively enlarged spleens, hand-assisted laparoscopic surgery (HALS) is a good supplement to laparoscopy, even if it offers an apparent contradiction to the philosophy of minimally invasive technique. HALS has been used increasingly in recent years in various areas of laparoscopy, and is a good alternative to open splenectomy in patients who have large spleens [35]. With HALS, the duration of surgery for large spleens can, in comparison with totally laparoscopic technique, be reduced by 30%, and the conversion rate by 8% [36].

Summary

Laparoscopy is a safe and effective technique for splenic surgery. It is the standard splenectomy method for normal to moderately enlarged spleens. With larger spleens, the hand-assisted technique can be an alternative to open splenectomy.

As in trauma surgery, more efforts toward splenic preservation should also be made in elective splenic surgery. We find that laparoscopic partial splenectomy is a safe method that is readily mastered. If the blood vessels are dissected carefully and in accordance with anatomical principles, hemisplenectomy can be done more quickly and with less blood loss than with open surgery.

References

[1] Pean J. Ovariotomie et splenotomie (Ovariectomy and splenectomy). 2nd edition. Paris: Germer-Bailliere; 1869. (in French)

[2] Morgenstern L. Evolution of splenic surgery: from mythology to modernity. Contemp Surg 1986;29:15.

[3] Morgenstern L, Rosenberger J, Geller SA. Tumors of the spleen. World J Surg 1985;9: 468–71.

[4] King H, Shumacker B. Splenic studies. Ann Surg 1952;136:239–46.

[5] Huntley CC. Infection following splenectomy in infants and children. Am J Dis Child 1958; 95:477–82.

[6] Singer DB. Postsplenectomy sepsis. In: Rosenberg HS, editor. Perspectives in pediatric pathology, vol. 1. Chicago: RP Bolande Year Book Medical Publishers; 1973. p. 295–307.

[7] Christo MC. Segmental resections of the spleen: report on the first eight cases operated on. O. Hospital (Rio) 1962;62:575–81.

[8] Morgenstern L. Subtotal splenectomy in myelofibrosis. Surgery 1966;60:336–9.

[9] Uranues S, Kronberger L, Kraft-Kine J. Partial splenic resection using the TA-stapler. Am J Surg 1994;168:49–53.

[10] Delaitre B. Splenectomy by the laparoscopic approach: report of a case. Presse Med 1991;20: 2263.

[11] Uranüs S, Pfeifer J, Schauer C, Kronberger L Jr, Rabl H, Ranftl G, et al. Laparoscopic partial splenic resection. Surg Laparosc Endosc 1995;5:133–6.

[12] Ziske CG. Partial splenectomy. Lancet 2002;359:1144.

[13] Ellison EC, Fabri PJ. Complications of splenectomy: etiology, prevention, and management. Surg Clin North Am 1983;63:1313–30.

[14] Green JB, Shackford SR, Sise MJ, Fridlund P. Late septic complications in adults following splenectomy for trauma: a prospective analysis in 144 patients. J Trauma 1986;26: 999–1003.

[15] Holdsworth RJ, Irving AD, Cushieri A. Postsplenectomy sepsis and its mortality rate: actual versus perceived risks. Br J Surg 1991;78:1031–8.

[16] West KW, Grosfeld JL. Postsplenectomy sepsis: historical background and current concepts. World J Surg 1985;9:477–83.

[17] Uranues S. Immunological functions. In: Uranues S, editor. Current spleen surgery. Munich (Germany): Zuckschwerdt; 1995. p. 12–4.

[18] Uranues S, Mischinger HJ, Pfeifer J, Kronberger L, Rabl H, Werkgartner G, et al. Hemostatic methods for the management of spleen and liver injuries. World J Surg 1996;20: 1107–12.

[19] Uranues S, Fingerhut A, Kronberger L, Pfeifer J, Mischinger HJ. Splenic trauma. European Surgery 1999;31:75–8.

[20] Thalhammer GH, Eber E, Uranues S, Pfeifer J, Zach MS. Partial splenectomy in cystic fibrosis patients with hypersplenism. Arch Dis Child 2003;88:143–6.
[21] Losanoff JE, Richman BW, Jones JW. Laparoscopic management of splenic cysts. Surg Laparosc Endosc Percutan Tech 2003;13:63–4.
[22] Morgenstern L. Nonparasitic splenic cysts: pathogenesis, classification, and treatment. J Am Coll Surg 2002;194:306–14.
[23] Seshadri PA, Poulin EC, Mamazza J, Schlachta CM. Technique for laparoscopic partial splenectomy. Surg Laparosc Endosc Percutan Tech 2000;10:106–9.
[24] Romano F, Caprotti R, Franciosi C, De Fina S, Colombo G, Uggeri F. Laparoscopic splenectomy using ligasure. Surg Endosc 2002;16:1608–11.
[25] Klingler A. Statistical methods in surgical research—a practical guide. European Surgery 2004;36(2):80–4.
[26] Wolf HM, Eibl MM, Georgi E, Samstag A, Spatz M, Uranüs S, Passl R. Long-term decrease of CD4 + CD45RA + T cells and impaired primary immune response after post-traumatic splenectomy. Br J Haematol 1999;107:55–68.
[27] Horowitz J, Smith JL, Weber TK, Rodriguez-Bigas MA, Petrelli NJ. Postoperative complications after splenectomy for hematologic malignancies. Ann Surg 1996;223:290–6.
[28] Schlachta CM, Poulin EC, Mamazza J. Laparoscopic splenectomy for hematologic malignancies. Surg Endosc 1999;13:865–8.
[29] Donini A, Baccarani U, Terrosu G, Corno V, Ermacora A, Pasqualucci A, et al. Laparoscopic vs open splenectomy in the management of hematologic diseases. Surg Endosc 1999;13:1220–5.
[30] Park A, Marcaccio M, Sternbach M, Witzke D, Fitzgerald P. Laparoscopic vs open splenectomy. Arch Surg 1999;134:1263–9.
[31] Heniford BT, Park A, Walsh RM, Kercher KW, Matthews BD, Frenette G, et al. Laparoscopic splenectomy in patients with normal-sized spleens versus splenomegaly: does size matter? Am Surg 2001;67:854–7.
[32] Baccarani U, Donini A, Terrosu G, Pasqualucci A, Bresadola F. Laparoscopic splenectomy for haematological diseases: review of current concepts and opinions. Eur J Surg 1999;165:917–23.
[33] Katkhouda N, Mavor E. Laparoscopic splenectomy. Surg Clin North Am 2000;80:1285–97.
[34] Uranues S. Laparoskopische Splenektomie (Laparoscopic splenectomy). Acta Chir Austriaca 2000;32:35–8.
[35] Targarona EM, Gracia E, Rodriguez M, Cerdan G, Balague C, Garriga J, et al. Hand-assisted laparoscopic surgery. Arch Surg 2003;138:133–41.
[36] Targarona EM, Balague C, Cerdan G, Espert JJ, Lacy AM, Visa J, et al. Hand-assisted laparoscopic splenectomy (HALS) in cases of splenomegaly. Surg Endosc 2002;16:426–30.

ELSEVIER
SAUNDERS

Surg Clin N Am 85 (2005) 91–103

SURGICAL
CLINICS OF
NORTH AMERICA

Laparoscopic repair of incisional hernias

William S. Cobb, MD, Kent W. Kercher, MD, B. Todd Heniford, MD*

Carolinas Laparoscopic and Advanced Surgery Program, Carolinas Medical Center,
1000 Blythe Boulevard, Charlotte, NC 28203, USA

One outcome of the greater than 2 million abdominal operations performed in the United States each year is an incisional hernia rate of 3% to 20% [1]. As a result, approximately 90,000 ventral hernia repairs are necessary annually. The increasing number of incisional hernias merely reflects the evolution of surgery, with the ability to perform larger abdominal operations such as aortic surgery and colectomy. Factors associated with formation of an incisional hernia include wound infection, morbid obesity, previous operations, immunosuppression, prostatism, and surgery for aortic aneurysmal disease. Abdominal wall defects typically occur within the first 5 years after the surgical incision is made, but may develop long afterward [2]. These hernias contribute greatly to the long-term morbidity of conventional surgery. Until techniques for the prevention of hernias are established, the repair of incisional hernias will remain an important concern to the general surgeon.

Several hernia repair methods have been described. Primary tissue repair using a "vest-over-pants" technique requires suture approximation of strong fascia on each side of the defect. Recurrence rates after this type of repair range from 31% to 54% during long-term follow-up [3,4]. The introduction of prosthetics revolutionized hernia surgery with the concept of a tension-free repair. The subsequent rate of recurrence has been lowered to less than 10% [5]; however; the required dissection of wide areas of soft tissue for mesh placement contributes to an increased incidence of wound infections and wound-related complications (12% or higher) [6–8]. These problems have stimulated a continuing search for new techniques for ventral herniorrhaphy.

---

* Corresponding author.
E-mail address: todd.heniford@carolinashealthcare.org (B.T. Heniford).

0039-6109/05/$ - see front matter © 2005 Elsevier Inc. All rights reserved.
doi:10.1016/j.suc.2004.09.006   surgical.theclinics.com

The laparoscopic repair of ventral hernias is rapidly evolving with patient and surgeon interest in less morbid herniorrhaphies and the appeal of minimally invasive surgery. The technique is based on the open, preperitoneal repair described by Stoppa [7] and Rives [9]. The placement of a large mesh in the preperitoneal location allows for an even distribution of forces along the surface area of the mesh, which may account for the strength of the repair and the decreased recurrence rates associated with it. The minimally invasive approach embraces the concept that a retromuscular mesh repair may be more durable, although the mesh is placed one layer deeper on an intact peritoneum compared with the open technique. The technique incorporates other fundamental components of the open repair, such as wide mesh overlap of the defect and the use of transabdominal fixation sutures to secure the mesh.

The feasibility of laparoscopic ventral hernia repair has been clearly established with large series of patients and good long-term follow-up [10–12]. The merit of the minimally invasive approach will be demonstrated with improved rates of recurrence, reduced risks of wound complications, and applicability of the technique for difficult patient populations.

Recurrence

The long term efficacy of any hernia repair depends on the rate of recurrence. As Sir Cecil Wakely stated in his presidential address to the Royal College of Surgeons in 1948, "A surgeon can do more for the community by operating on hernia cases and seeing that his recurrence rate is low than he can by operating on cases of malignant disease [13]." The use of prosthetics and a reduced rate of recurrence have clearly been demonstrated for defects larger than 4 cm in diameter. In a prospective study evaluating primary tissue repair, Luijendijk and colleagues [4] showed unacceptable 5-year cumulative recurrence rates of 44% and 73% for midline hernias measuring 3 to 6 cm and 6 to 12 cm, respectively. Hesselink and associates [2] confirmed that incisional hernias larger than 4 cm had a significantly higher recurrence rate than smaller defects (41% versus 25%). They concluded that hernias larger than 4 cm in diameter should be repaired with prosthetics. The repair of incisional hernias with mesh has dramatically reduced the number of recurrences when compared with open repair [14].

The rate of recurrence following any hernia repair depends on the technique used for repair. One of the most critical technical points of the laparoscopic repair that may significantly impact the rate of recurrence is adequate mesh fixation. The most widespread technique in laparoscopic ventral hernia repair involves fixation of the mesh with tacks and transabdominal permanent sutures [10]. Some surgeons have tried to reduce operating time and possibly postoperative discomfort by eliminating the use of transabdominal sutures completely, or by markedly reducing the number of sutures used and leaning primarily on the use of a laparoscopic tacker. In an attempt to decrease postoperative suture site pain, Berger and colleagues [15] used sutures to orient the mesh for tacking and did not tie them. With this technique, their recurrence rate is 2.7% (4/147) at a mean follow-up of 15 months. Carbajo and associates [12] have the largest series without suture fixation. Over an 8-year period, 270 repairs were performed using two layers of tacks to fix the mesh, or a "double-crown" technique. With an average follow-up of 44 months, there were 12 recurrences (4.4%). In another multi-institutional series [16], 100 consecutive patients underwent laparoscopic ventral hernia repair without suture fixation. There was a single recurrence (1%) over follow-up ranging from 1 to 60 months. Bageacu et al [17] reported 19 recurrences that were detected on examination and confirmed with CT scan in 121 patients (15.7%) over a mean follow-up of 49 months. The study authors attributed their recurrence rate to inadequate mesh fixation with metallic tacks alone. Other series have attributed early failures to inadequate tack fixation alone, and the investigators have since added additional transabdominal sutures to their technique [11,18,19].

The physics of mesh fixation during laparoscopic ventral hernia repair do not support the sole placement of tacks. The majority of the meshes used for laparoscopic ventral hernia repair are roughly 1 mm thick, and the spiral tacks used are 4-mm long and take up a 1-mm profile on the surface of the patch. A perfectly placed tack can be expected to penetrate only 2 mm beyond the mesh; hence, tacks will likely not give the same holding strength as a full-thickness abdominal wall suture. Because many candidates presenting for laparoscopic ventral hernia repair are obese (having a substantial amount of preperitoneal fat), the 2-mm purchase of the tack will not reach the fascia in most cases. Furthermore, the mesh is placed against the peritoneum, so any ingrowth of the mesh is most likely into the peritoneum and not into fascia.

Experimental studies have confirmed the superior strength of sutures versus tacks alone in mesh fixation to the abdominal wall. The authors' group has specifically examined the strength of full-thickness trans-abdominal suture versus two commercially available metallic fixation devices in an animal model. In these studies, the initial fixation strength for suture materials, both absorbable and permanent, was significantly greater than for either the metallic tack or anchor device; however, absorbable sutures showed a significant loss of strength at 8 weeks when compared with permanent sutures [20]. Van't Riet and coauthors [21] demonstrated in a porcine model that the tensile strength of sutures in transabdominal mesh is 2.5 times greater than that of tacks. If the mesh remains where it is placed, assuming adequate overlap of the defect, the rate of recurrence should be zero. Therefore, the authors believe that suture fixation of the mesh in laparoscopic ventral hernia repair is imperative, especially during the early period of mesh incorporation.

As with the retromuscular, sublay repair described by Stoppa [7], Rives et al [9], and Wantz [22], the laparoscopic repair of ventral defects capitalizes on the physics of Pascal's principle of hydrostatics by using the forces that create the hernia defect to hold the mesh in place (Fig. 1). The amount of adequate coverage for mesh repair of hernias is not known. It stands to reason that a wide overlap of the defect with mesh would help to counteract the intra-abdominal forces from displacing the mesh into the defect. The laparoscopic technique allows for easier placement of a prosthesis with good overlap. In the open approach, attaining an overlap of 3 to 5 cm requires extensive soft-tissue dissection, with the resultant increase in wound complications. Larger defects should require more overlap, and smaller "Swiss-cheese" defects theoretically need less. Most authors advocate an overlap of at least 3 cm. More overlap (5 cm) is recommended in patients with increased risk of recurrence, such as the morbidly obese and those who have large defects [10,19].

Another recognized cause of recurrence following ventral hernia repair is a missed hernia. The laparoscopic approach affords the surgeon the ability to clearly and definitively define the margins of the hernia defect and to identify additional defects that may not have been clinically apparent preoperatively. Complete visualization of the fascia underlying the previous incision allows for identification of smaller "Swiss-cheese" defects that could be missed in an open approach [23].

In a review of the recent larger series with mean follow-up more than 12 months, the overall rate of recurrence for laparoscopic ventral hernia repair is 4.3% (Table 1). There are eight series in which only tacks or the initial cardinal sutures were used for mesh fixation, and the recurrence is 5.6%. When the technique uses transabdominal sutures, the reported recurrence rate is 3.8%. It is difficult to compare the two techniques with regard to recurrence without a randomized, prospective trial. This study, however, will be difficult to perform due to the strong opinions that most laparoscopists have regarding the use of sutures. Other factors contributing to recurrence, such as prior failed attempts at repair, obesity, and degree of mesh overlap would need to be controlled as much as possible.

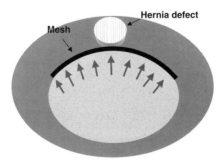

Fig. 1. Pascal's principle—wide mesh overlap of defect distributes pressure equally over larger surface area.

Table 1
Rate of recurrence in select series of laparoscopic ventral hernia repair with and without the use of suture fixation

Name	Year	n	Defect size (cm^2)	Mesh overlap	Suture fixation	Recurrence	Mean F/U (mths)
Franklin [11]	2004	384	NR	3–5 cm	"Most cases"[a]	11 (2.9%)	47.1
LeBlanc [19]	2003	200	111	≥3 cm	Yes	13 (6.5%)	36
Bower [28]	2003	100	124.4	≥3 cm	Yes	2 (2%)	6.5
Eid [18]	2003	23	103	3–5 cm	Yes[b]	0	13
Heniford [10]	2003	850	118	≥3–5 cm	Yes	40 (4.7%)	20.2
Raftopoulos [37]	2002	50	124.6	2–4 cm	Yes	1 (2.0%)	NR
Ben-Haim [38]	2002	100	30[d]	NR	Yes	2 (2.0%)	19
Berger [15]	2002	150	96, 83[e]	3–5 cm	Yes	4 (3.0%)	15
Aura [39]	2002	86	26.5[d]	5 cm	Yes	6 (7.0%)	37
Parker [40]	2002	50	206	4 cm	Yes	0	41
Birgisson [34]	2001	64	4–416	≥3 cm	Yes	0	1–35
Total		2057				79 (3.8%)	
Sanchez [41]	2004	85	69	4–5 cm	No	3 (3.5%)	20
Eid [18]	2003	56	103	3–5 cm	No[a]	4 (5.0%)	34
Carbajo [12]	2003	270	145	5 cm	No	12 (4.4%)	44
Bencini [42]	2003	50	NR	≥4 cm	No[c]	1 (2.0%)	14
Bageacu [17]	2002	159	1–314[d]	5 cm	No[a]	19 (11.9%)	49
Gillian [16]	2002	100	NR	3–5 cm	No	1 (1.0%)	1–60
Kirshtein [43]	2002	103	175	≥3 cm	No[a,c]	4 (4.0%)	26
Kua [44]	2002	21	NR	2–3 cm	No	3 (14.3%)	12
Total		844				47 (5.6%)	
Overall		2901				126 (4.3%)	

Abbreviations: F/U, follow-up; mths, months; NR, not reported.
[a] Authors cited omission of transabdominal suture in cause of recurrence.
[b] Sutures used in last 6 months of study.
[c] Initial cardinal sutures used only with tacks.
[d] Calculated.
[e] Primary and secondary defect sizes, respectively.

Mesh infection

One of the greatest benefits of the laparoscopic approach to incisional hernias is the reduction in wound and mesh infectious complications. The open technique of ventral hernia repair has historically been associated with a high rate of cellulitis and mesh infection. In his landmark article, Dr. Stoppa [7] experienced a "wound sepsis" rate of 12%. Wound problems are not unexpected, due to the large amount of soft-tissue dissection required for retromuscular placement of large pieces of mesh. Placing the mesh intra-abdominally through a trocar, however, obviates the need for extensive tissue dissection that potentially devascularizes the fascia and causes hematoma formation, both of which contribute to wound and mesh complications.

Mesh infection remains a serious complication associated with laparoscopic ventral hernia repair. Although the incidence is very low, the consequences are severe. Skin pathogens are responsible for most mesh infections. Every effort is made to avoid contact of the mesh with the skin. The use of an iodine-impregnated, adhesive drape on the abdomen can help accomplish this goal. Infections of polypropylene meshes can be managed locally with surgical drainage and excision of exposed, unincorporated segments. Meshes containing expanded polytetrafluoroethylene (ePTFE) require removal of the prosthetic material in most cases. There is one reported success with local drainage of ePTFE and placement of a vacuum-assisted wound device [24]. Removal of mesh results in return of the defect and its added morbidity. Early experiments with antibiotic impregnated mesh are encouraging, and indicate that its use may lead to fewer mesh infections. In one study, the in-vitro susceptibility to infection with *Staphylococcus aureus* was evaluated for various prosthetic and biologic meshes. The biomaterials tested were DualMesh Plus (W.L. Gore and Associates, Flagstaff, Arizona), which is ePTFE impregnated with silver/chlorhexidine, DualMesh (ePTFE; W.L. Gore and Associates, Flagstaff, Arizona), Marlex (polypropylene; C.R. Bard, Inc., Murray Hill, New Jersey), Composix (ePTFE and polypropylene; C.R. Bard, Inc., Murray Hill, New Jersey), SepraMesh (Genzyme Corporation, Cambridge, Massachusetts), Surgisis (Cook, Surgical Inc., Bloomington, Indiana), and AlloDerm (Lifecell Corporation, Branchburg, New Jersey). Impregnation of ePTFE with silver/chlorhexidine killed all the inoculated bacteria, preventing their proliferation on the mesh surface [25].

A compilation of the reported series with at least 50 patients is demonstrated in Table 2. The mesh infection rate was 20 per 3276 cases, or 0.6%. Cellulitis of the trocar sites that resolved with antibiotics occurred in 35 cases, or 1.1%. When including all wound and mesh complications, the rate of occurrence is 1.7%. This percentage compares favorably with the 12% to 18% rate of wound complications reported with the open prosthetic repair series [7,8,26,27]. Again, the most compelling argument for the laparoscopic approach to incisional hernias is the minimization of soft-tissue dissection and the associated reduction in the morbidity associated with local wound complications and in the potential for infection of the implanted mesh.

Seroma formation

Seroma formation is not unique to the laparoscopic approach. Most seromas develop above the mesh and within the retained hernia sac. The majority of patients form seromas postoperatively, but they typically resolve spontaneously without intervention. Berger and associates [15] performed

Table 2
Wound and mesh complications in large series of laparoscopic ventral hernia repairs (≥50 patients)

Name	Year	# pts	Seroma	Mesh infection	Wound infection	Fistula
Sanchez [41]	2004	85	8	0	0	0
Franklin [11]	2004	384	12	1	3	0
LeBlanc [19]	2003	200	15	4	0	0
Bower [28]	2003	100	1	2	0	0
Eid [18]	2003	79	3	0	0	0
Bencini [42]	2003	50	8	0	0	0
Carbajo [12]	2003	270	32	0	0	1
Rosen [45]	2003	100	4	2	4	0
Heniford [10]	2003	850	21	6	9	0
Bageacu [17]	2002	159	22	0	4	2
Aura [39]	2002	86	2	0	0	0
Raftopoulos [37]	2002	50	7	1	2	0
Ben-Haim [38]	2002	100	11	0	0	0
Gillian [16]	2002	100	3	0	0	0
Kirshtein [43]	2002	103	"most"	2	3	0
Berger [15]	2002	150	139	0	0	0
Birgisson [34]	2001	64	3	0	2	0
Chowbey [46]	2000	202	49	0	5	0
Toy [47]	1998	144	23	2	3	0
Overall		3276	363 (11.4%)	20 (0.6%)	35 (1.1%)	3 (0.1%)

ultrasound examinations on 139 of 150 patients postoperatively following laparoscopic ventral hernia repair, and found a seroma or hematoma in all patients studied. The rate of seroma formation in reported series varies depending on when the investigators evaluate for it. The mean incidence of seroma at a range of 4 to 8 weeks is 11.4% in the large reported series (see Table 2). In the largest multi-institutional trial, seromas that were clinically apparent more than 8 weeks postoperatively were considered a complication and occurred 2.6% of the time [10]. Regardless of whether they are aspirated under sterile conditions or allowed to resolve, seromas rarely result in long-term problems. It is imperative that surgeons inform their patients preoperatively about the likelihood of a seroma and that, if one becomes clinically evident after surgery, it will be managed expectantly unless it causes discomfort or becomes persistent. Large seromas are fortunately uncommon; however, they can place tension on the skin, causing necrosis with the associated risk of mesh infection. Aspiration is recommended for seromas that enlarge or persist before they reach these extremes [10].

Persistent pain

After laparoscopic ventral hernia repair, patients will occasionally complain of persistent pain and point tenderness at a transabdominal suture site. Transabdominal suture site pain after laparoscopic ventral hernia repair is not uncommon and occurs in 1% to 3% of patients in the reported series of repairs using transabdominal sutures [10,11,19,28]. Interestingly, in the larger series not using transabdominal fixation, postoperative abdominal pain is reported by 25.6% of the patients [12], with persistent pain occurring in 7.4% of cases [16].

The discomfort at the transabdominal fixation suture sites typically resolves within 6 to 8 weeks [29]. Over the short-term, this can be problematic, and little is understood as to reasons it occurs. A possible explanation may be that the transabdominal suture entraps an intercostal nerve as it courses through the abdominal muscles. Local muscle ischemia may be another possibility. The first line of treatment can be a course of oral nonsteroidal anti-inflammatory therapy or simply additional time. If the pain persists, injecting local anesthetic at these painful suture sites has good results. The transabdominal suture site is injected circumferentially with 25 to 30 mL of 0.25% bupivacaine with 1:200,000 epinephrine and 1% lidocaine at the level of the abdominal musculature, using a blunted 22-gauge needle. The needle is blunted so the surgeon can feel the tip of the needle penetrate the anterior fascia. In a study conducted by the authors, the majority (92%) of patients undergoing treatment with an injection had complete relief of their symptoms [30]. Most of those responding to therapy (91%) required only a single injection. This is perhaps due to the ability to block the afferent signal temporarily and allow the hypersensitivity to subside [30].

Morbid obesity

The morbidly obese population represents a significant portion of the patients that present for repair of a ventral hernia. Obesity has been clearly established as a risk factor for development of incisional hernias. Sugerman and colleagues [31] reported that severe obesity (body mass index $\geq$35 kg/m^2) was a greater risk factor for incisional hernia and recurrence than chronic steroid use. This group has shown that severely obese patients, and especially those with central obesity, have increased intra-abdominal pressure [32]. This higher pressure creates more strain on the mesh placed for the hernia repair, which is probably responsible for the increased incidence of incisional hernia and rate of recurrence following repair. The laparoscopic approach is ideal in the obese patient, due to the smaller wounds and theoretically, decreased wound complications [33].

Complications of ventral herniorrhaphy, such as wound infection and recurrence, are elevated in the obese population. Laparoscopic ventral hernia repair can be safely performed in the morbidly obese patient. The morbidly obese (body mass index $\geq$40) have significantly longer operative times, larger hernia defects, and higher rates of recurrence. Over a 9-year period, Heniford and associates [10] demonstrated that this population was nearly four times more likely to have a recurrence after laparoscopic ventral hernia repair (7.8% versus 2.0%). Birgisson et al [34] reported an increase in operative times and defect sizes as well. In their experience, 16 patients who had a body mass index ≥ 40 had five minor complications (31%), but no major complications or recurrences at a mean of 8.5 months.

Previous failed repairs

The laparoscopic approach is an excellent choice for recurrent hernias that have failed prior attempts at repair. Laparoscopic entry into the peritoneal cavity avoids dissection through the previous operative site. This technique is ideal for patients who have failed preperitoneal or onlay repairs using prosthetics, because the dissection avoids disrupting these meshes and risking infection. The "battlefield abdomen" that has had numerous failed repairs and several pieces of mesh complicated by infection may be better served by an open repair, however. Multiple defects resulting in the "Swiss cheese" abdomen are well suited for laparoscopic hernioplasty. The intra-abdominal view better identifies all of the defects and allows for better prosthetic coverage.

Patients who have failed prior open attempts at repair demonstrate significantly longer operative times (134 minutes versus 111 minutes). Those who have had previous repairs have a higher rate of complications (17.8% versus 10.4%), and a greater than three times increased risk of hernia recurrence (7.1% versus 2.3%). The rate of conversions to open surgery is not different [10]. Patients who have failed open repairs and previously placed intra-abdominal mesh frequently present for laparoscopic repair. In the larger series, those who have prior repairs range from 21% to 34% [10,12,19], and the number of previous repairs ranges from 1 to 11 [10]. These patients are more technically challenging, but they can be safely treated with a laparoscopic approach to their recurrent defect.

Minimally invasive versus open approaches

Several reports have touted the benefits of the laparoscopic approach versus the open technique for ventral hernia repair with regard to postoperative pain, morbidity, length of stay, and wound complications. Many studies have been conducted and published in both Europe and North America. The results of these studies point to laparoscopic ventral hernia repair as having reduced perioperative morbidity and reduced rates of hernia recurrence during follow-up [10,19]. A small number of studies comparing laparoscopic ventral hernia repair and the open procedure directly have been conducted; however, the number of patients has been small, the studies have not been randomized, and much of the data have not been prospective [23,33,35,36,48–53]. Nonetheless, these studies reliably show that laparoscopic ventral hernia repair has advantages over the open hernia repair, in that it has fewer perioperative complications, a reduced hospital stay, and fewer hernia recurrences.

Only two prospective studies comparing laparoscopic ventral hernia repair with open hernia repair have been published in the literature. These studies, conducted by Carbajo et al [35] and DeMaria et al [34], support the advantages purported by the literature from the noncomparative studies previously mentioned. Carbajo et al [35] randomly assigned 60 patients to receive either laparoscopic ventral hernia repair or the open procedure. The two groups were fairly similar in that they did not differ significantly in incisional hernia type, size of defect, age, or sex distribution. Postoperative hospital stay and operative time were significantly shorter in the laparoscopic ventral hernia repair group; however, it should be noted that Carbajo and colleagues did not use transabdominal wall sutures to secure the mesh, which likely contributed to reduced operating time. They also reported that the laparoscopic ventral hernia repair group had fewer complications and a reduced hernia recurrence rate (0% versus 6.7%) during their 27 month follow-up period. DeMaria and associates [36] prospectively compared laparoscopic and open ventral hernia repairs at a tertiary, university setting. There were 39 consecutive patients in their study. The decision on the surgical approach was made by the attending surgeon, and more recurrent repairs were treated laparoscopically. Ninety percent of the laparoscopic group were treated on an outpatient basis, compared with only 7% in the open group. The incidence of complications and the rate of recurrence were not different between the two groups.

Based on the data from the comparative studies (Table 3), postoperative complications are less in the laparoscopic group (23.2% versus 30.2%). The incidence of wound and mesh infections is lower in the laparoscopic patients as well. In the numerous series of open and laparoscopic ventral hernia

Table 3
Comparison studies of laparoscopic and open ventral hernia repairs

Name	Year	# patients lap / open		Morbidity lap / open		Mesh infection lap / open		Wound infection lap / open		Recurrence lap / open	
McGreevy [48]	2003	65	71	5	15	2	0	0	7	—	—
Raftopoulos [49]	2003	50	22	14	10	1	0	1	1	1	4
Wright [50]	2002	90	90	15	31	1	1	1	8	1	5
Robbins [51]	2001	18	31	—	—	1	4	1	0	—	—
DeMaria [36]	2000	21	18	13	13	1	2	1	4	1	0
Chari [52]	2000	14	14	2	2	0	1	—	—	—	—
Carbajo [35]	1999	30	30	20	6	0	3	0	5	1	2
Ramshaw [33]	1999	79	174	15	46	1	5	6	2	2	36
Park [23]	1998	56	49	10	18	2	1	0	2	6	17
Holzman [53]	1997	21	16	5	5	0	1	1	0	2	2
Percent				23.2	30.2	2.0	3.5	2.6	5.8	4.0	16.5

repairs (see Table 3), the recurrence rate is 4.0% for the laparoscopic approach and 16.5% for the open technique. The long-term follow-up data from the larger laparoscopic series continue to demonstrate the superiority of potential advantages over the procedure when compared with the open approach [10,19]. The authors believe that the time for prospective, randomized studies comparing laparoscopic with open ventral hernia repair has passed. With the numerous cases touting low rates of mesh infection and recurrence with the minimally invasive approach, it would be difficult and potentially unethical to recruit patients for such a study.

Summary

Laparoscopic repair of incisional hernias results in a low rate of conversion to open surgery, a short hospital stay, and an acceptable overall complication rate. Additionally, the procedure results in extremely low risk of infection and a low risk of recurrence. The laparoscopic approach appears to be effective in complex patients, especially those who are obese and who have had failed prior open repairs. With sufficient long-term follow-up to support the durability of the procedure, laparoscopic ventral hernia repair should be considered the standard of care.

References

[1] Read RC, Yoder G. Recent trends in the management of incisional herniation. Arch Surg 1989;124(4):485–8.
[2] Hesselink VJ, Luijendijk RW, de Wilt JH, et al. An evaluation of risk factors in incisional hernia recurrence. Surg Gynecol Obstet 1993;176(3):228–34.
[3] Anthony T, Bergen PC, Kim LT, et al. Factors affecting recurrence following incisional herniorrhaphy. World J Surg 2000;24(1):95–100 [discussion: 101].
[4] Luijendijk RW, Lemmen MH, Hop WC, et al. Incisional hernia recurrence following "vest-over-pants" or vertical Mayo repair of primary hernias of the midline. World J Surg 1997; 21(1):62–5 [discussion: 66].
[5] Liakakos T, Karanikas I, Panagiotidis H, et al. Use of Marlex mesh in the repair of recurrent incisional hernia. Br J Surg 1994;81(2):248–9.
[6] Leber GE, Garb JL, Alexander AI, et al. Long-term complications associated with prosthetic repair of incisional hernias. Arch Surg 1998;133(4):378–82.
[7] Stoppa RE. The treatment of complicated groin and incisional hernias. World J Surg 1989; 13(5):545–54.
[8] White TJ, Santos MC, Thompson JS. Factors affecting wound complications in repair of ventral hernias. Am Surg 1998;64(3):276–80.
[9] Rives J, Pire JC, Flament JB, et al. Le traitment des grandes eventrations: nouvelle indication thérapeutiques. A propos de 322 cas. [Treatment of large eventrations. New therapeutic indications apropos of 322 cases]. Chirurgie 1985;111(3):215–25.
[10] Heniford BT, Park A, Ramshaw BJ, et al. Laparoscopic repair of ventral hernias: nine years' experience with 850 consecutive hernias. Ann Surg 2003;238(3):391–9 [discussion: 399–400].
[11] Franklin ME Jr, Gonzalez JJ Jr, Glass JL, et al. Laparoscopic ventral and incisional hernia repair: an 11-year experience. Hernia 2004;8(1):23–7.

[12] Carbajo MA, Martp del Olmo JC, Blanco JI, et al. Laparoscopic approach to incisional hernia. Surg Endosc 2003;17(1):118–22.
[13] Wakely C. Presidential address. British Hernia Centre, London, England, Available at: http://www.hernia.org/recurrent.html. Accessed October 15, 2004.
[14] Luijendijk RW, Hop WC, van den Tol MP, et al. A comparison of suture repair with mesh repair for incisional hernia. N Engl J Med 2000;343(6):392–8.
[15] Berger D, Bientzle M, Muller A. Postoperative complications after laparoscopic incisional hernia repair. Incidence and treatment. Surg Endosc 2002;16(12):1720–3.
[16] Gillian GK, Geis WP, Grover G. Laparoscopic incisional and ventral hernia repair (LIVH): an evolving outpatient technique. JSLS 2002;6(4):315–22.
[17] Bageacu S, Blanc P, Breton C, et al. Laparoscopic repair of incisional hernia: a retrospective study of 159 patients. Surg Endosc 2002;16(2):345–8.
[18] Eid GM, Prince JM, Mattar SG, et al. Medium-term follow-up confirms the safety and durability of laparoscopic ventral hernia repair with PTFE. Surgery 2003;134(4):599–603 [discussion: 603–4].
[19] LeBlanc KA, Whitaker JM, Bellanger DE, et al. Laparoscopic incisional and ventral hernioplasty: lessons learned from 200 patients. Hernia 2003;7(3):118–24.
[20] Joels CS, Matthews BD, Austin CE, et al. Evaluation of fixation strength and adhesion formation after ePTFE mesh placement with various fixation devices. Presented at SAGES Scientific Session. Denver, Colorado, April 2, 2004.
[21] van't Riet M, de Vos van Steenwijk PJ, Kleinrensink GJ, et al. Tensile strength of mesh fixation methods in laparoscopic incisional hernia repair. Surg Endosc 2002;16(12):1713–6.
[22] Wantz GE. Giant prosthetic reinforcement of the visceral sac. Surg Gynecol Obstet 1989; 169(5):408–17.
[23] Park A, Birch DW, Lovrics P. Laparoscopic and open incisional hernia repair: a comparison study. Surgery 1998;124(4):816–21 [discussion: 821–2].
[24] Kercher KW, Sing RF, Matthews BD, et al. Successful salvage of infected PTFE mesh after ventral hernia repair. Ostomy Wound Manage 2002;48(10):40–2; 44–5.
[25] Carbonell AM, Matthews BD, Dreau D, et al. An in-vitro study of susceptibility to infection of various prosthetic mesh biomaterials. Presented at International Hernia Congress. London, June 19, 2003.
[26] Rios A, Rodriguez JM, Munitiz V, et al. Factors that affect recurrence after incisional herniorrhaphy with prosthetic material. Eur J Surg 2001;167(11):855–9.
[27] McLanahan D, King LT, Weems C, et al. Retrorectus prosthetic mesh repair of midline abdominal hernia. Am J Surg 1997;173(5):445–9.
[28] Bower CE, Reade CC, Kirby LW, et al. Complications of laparoscopic incisional-ventral hernia repair: the experience of a single institution. Surg Endosc 2004;18(4):672–5.
[29] Heniford BT, Park A, Ramshaw BJ, et al. Laparoscopic ventral and incisional hernia repair in 407 patients. J Am Coll Surg 2000;190(6):645–50.
[30] Carbonell AM, Harold KL, Mahmutovic AJ, et al. Local injection for the treatment of suture site pain after laparoscopic ventral hernia repair. Am Surg 2003;69(8):688–91 [discussion: 691–2].
[31] Sugerman HJ, Kellum JM Jr, Reines HD, et al. Greater risk of incisional hernia with morbidly obese than steroid-dependent patients and low recurrence with prefascial poly-propylene mesh. Am J Surg 1996;171(1):80–4.
[32] Sugerman H, Windsor A, Bessos M, et al. Effects of surgically induced weight loss on urinary bladder pressure, sagittal abdominal diameter and obesity co-morbidity. Int J Obes Relat Metab Disord 1998;22(3):230–5.
[33] Ramshaw BJ, Esartia P, Schwab J, et al. Comparison of laparoscopic and open ventral herniorrhaphy. Am Surg 1999;65(9):827–31 [discussion: 831–2].
[34] Birgisson G, Park AE, Mastrangelo MJ Jr, et al. Obesity and laparoscopic repair of ventral hernias. Surg Endosc 2001;15(12):1419–22.

[35] Carbajo MA, Martin del Olmo JC, Blanco JI, et al. Laparoscopic treatment vs open surgery in the solution of major incisional and abdominal wall hernias with mesh. Surg Endosc 1999; 13(3):250–2.

[36] DeMaria EJ, Moss JM, Sugerman HJ. Laparoscopic intraperitoneal polytetrafluoro-ethylene (PTFE) prosthetic patch repair of ventral hernia. Prospective comparison to open prefascial polypropylene mesh repair. Surg Endosc 2000;14(4):326–9.

[37] Raftopoulos I, Vanuno D, Khorsand J, et al. Outcome of laparoscopic ventral hernia repair in correlation with obesity, type of hernia, and hernia size. J Laparoendosc Adv Surg Tech A 2002;12(6):425–9.

[38] Ben-Haim M, Kuriansky J, Tal R, et al. Pitfalls and complications with laparoscopic intraperitoneal expanded polytetrafluoroethylene patch repair of postoperative ventral hernia. Surg Endosc 2002;16(5):785–8.

[39] Aura T, Habib E, Mekkaoui M, et al. Laparoscopic tension-free repair of anterior abdominal wall incisional and ventral hernias with an intraperitoneal Gore-Tex mesh: prospective study and review of the literature. J Laparoendosc Adv Surg Tech A 2002;12(4): 263–7.

[40] Parker HH 3rd, Nottingham JM, Bynoe RP, et al. Laparoscopic repair of large incisional hernias. Am Surg 2002;68(6):530–3 [discussion: 533–4].

[41] Sanchez LJ, Bencini L, Moretti R. Recurrences after laparoscopic ventral hernia repair: results and critical review. Hernia 2004;8(2):138–43.

[42] Bencini L, Sanchez LJ, Scatizzi M, et al. Laparoscopic treatment of ventral hernias: prospective evaluation. Surg Laparosc Endosc Percutan Tech 2003;13(1):16–9.

[43] Kirshtein B, Lantsberg L, Avinoach E, et al. Laparoscopic repair of large incisional hernias. Surg Endosc 2002;16(12):1717–9.

[44] Kua KB, Coleman M, Martin I, et al. Laparoscopic repair of ventral incisional hernia. ANZ J Surg 2002;72(4):296–9.

[45] Rosen M, Brody F, Ponsky J, et al. Recurrence after laparoscopic ventral hernia repair. Surg Endosc 2003;17(1):123–8.

[46] Chowbey PK, Sharma A, Khullar R, et al. Laparoscopic ventral hernia repair. J Lap-aroendosc Adv Surg Tech A 2000;10(2):79–84.

[47] Toy FK, Bailey RW, Carey S, et al. Prospective, multicenter study of laparoscopic ventral hernioplasty. Preliminary results. Surg Endosc 1998;12(7):955–9.

[48] McGreevy JM, Goodney PP, Birkmeyer CM, et al. A prospective study comparing the complication rates between laparoscopic and open ventral hernia repairs. Surg Endosc 2003; 17(11):1778–80.

[49] Raftopoulos I, Vanuno D, Khorsand J, et al. Comparison of open and laparoscopic prosthetic repair of large ventral hernias. JSLS 2003;7(3):227–32.

[50] Wright BE, Niskanen BD, Peterson DJ, et al. Laparoscopic ventral hernia repair: are there comparative advantages over traditional methods of repair? Am Surg 2002;68(3):291–5 [discussion: 295–6].

[51] Robbins SB, Pofahl WE, Gonzalez RP. Laparoscopic ventral hernia repair reduces wound complications. Am Surg 2001;67(9):896–900.

[52] Chari R, Chari V, Eisenstat M, et al. A case controlled study of laparoscopic incisional hernia repair. Surg Endosc 2000;14(2):117–9.

[53] Holzman MD, Purut CM, Reintgen K, et al. Laparoscopic ventral and incisional hernioplasty. Surg Endosc 1997;11(1):32–5.

ELSEVIER
SAUNDERS

SURGICAL
CLINICS OF
NORTH AMERICA

Surg Clin N Am 85 (2005) 105–118

Laparoscopic repair of paraesophageal hernia

Dave R. Lal, MD, Carlos A. Pellegrini, MD*,
Brant K. Oelschlager, MD

*Department of Surgery, Center for Videoendoscopic Surgery, University of Washington
Medical Center, 959 NE Pacific Street, Box 356410, Seattle, WA 98195, USA*

Management and treatment of patients who have paraesophageal hernia (PEH) has undergone a transformation since its first description by Akerlund in 1926 [1]. For nearly 20 years, surgical teaching had dictated that patients who have PEH undergo surgical correction at diagnosis to avoid potential complications of gastric bleeding, strangulation, or perforation [2,3]. Over the last decade, this dictum has come under scrutiny [4]. With recent studies better defining the natural history of PEH, asymptomatic patients may be treated in a conservative manner. This is especially true in the often elderly patient who has multiple comorbidities and is referred for surgical management of an asymptomatic PEH.

Further controversy exists concerning the best surgical approach for repair (laparoscopic versus open), the presence and management of short esophagus, the need for prosthetic reinforcement of the hiatus, and the need for fundoplication. This article addresses each of these points with a review of the associated literature.

Definition

Hiatal hernias are classified as one of the following four types:

Type I: The gastroesophageal junction migrates through the hiatus (Fig. 1). This is commonly referred to as a sliding hiatal hernia and may predispose the patient to reflux.

* Corresponding author.
E-mail address: pellegri@u.washington.edu (C.A. Pellegrini).

0039-6109/05/$ - see front matter © 2005 Elsevier Inc. All rights reserved.
doi:10.1016/j.suc.2004.09.008
surgical.theclinics.com

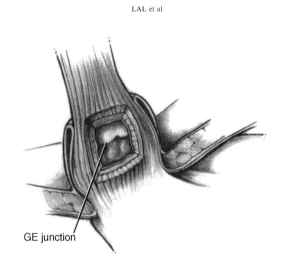

GE junction

Fig. 1. Type I hiatal hernia is also called a sliding hernia. (*From* Townsend CM, Beauchamp RD, Evers BM, et al, editors. Sabiston textbook of surgery—the biological basis of modern surgical practice. 17th edition. Philadelphia: WB Saunders; 2004. p. 1153; with permission.)

Type II: The gastric fundus herniates through the hiatus with the gastroesophageal junction maintaining its normal intra-abdominal position (Fig. 2). This true paraesophageal hernia is rare and is referred to as a rolling hiatal hernia.

Type III: The gastric fundus and gastroesophageal junction herniate through the hiatus into the thorax (Fig. 3). This represents a combination of Types I and II.

Type IV: A Type III hernia with the addition of other organs (eg, spleen, colon, omentum) herniating through the hiatus into the thorax.

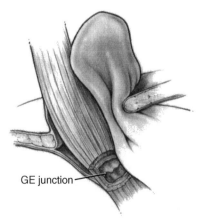

GE junction

Fig. 2. Type II hiatal hernia is also known as a rolling hernia. (*From* Townsend CM, Beauchamp RD, Evers BM, et al, editors. Sabiston textbook of surgery—the biological basis of modern surgical practice. 17th edition. Philadelphia: WB Saunders; 2004. p. 1153; with permission.)

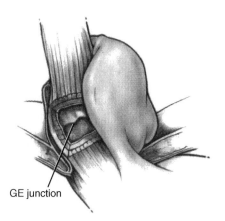

GE junction

Fig. 3. Type III hiatal hernia is referred to as a mixed hernia. (*From* Townsend CM, Beauchamp RD, Evers BM, et al, editors. Sabiston textbook of surgery—the biological basis of modern surgical practice. 17th edition. Philadelphia: WB Saunders; 2004. p. 1153; with permission.)

Etiology

Although the precise etiology of PEH is unknown, the current theory is that PEH results from progression of a hiatal hernia. Hiatal hernias are more common in younger patients and are seven times more common than PEH [5]. Progressive weakening and stretching of the phrenoesophageal membrane and concomitant weakening and enlargement of the diaphragmatic hiatus are key factors in PEH formation. This scenario allows progressive herniation of the stomach into the posterior mediastinum. Increased intra-abdominal pressure also encourages progression of PEH formation. These theories are given strength by the increased incidence of PEH in the elderly population. Also, conditions leading to increased intra-abdominal pressure, such as chronic obstructive pulmonary disease, asthma, obesity, chronic constipation, and heavy physical labor, are risk factors for formation of PEH.

In some cases, herniation of the stomach into the mediastinum may result in potentially devastating complications of gastric incarceration or volvulus. Since the sentinel articles by Skinner and Belsey [3] and Hill [2] describing the high morbidity and mortality associated with these complications, an aggressive surgical approach has been advocated. Historically, the incidence of developing a catastrophic complication has been estimated too be as high as 29%. This was reported in 1967, when 21 asymptomatic patients were treated nonoperatively for PEH, and 6 went on to develop strangulation, perforation, or significant bleeding [3]. Recent papers have documented a much lower incidence. Allen et al [6] followed 23 PEH patients for a median of 78 months, with none developing gastric complications. Stylopoulos and coworkers [7] created a decision analytical model to determine if asymptomatic PEH patients benefit from elective laparoscopic PEH repair. A computer model was created examining 5 million patients aged 65 years or older. Using published studies, mortality, recurrence, and progression rates were determined. In reviewing 21 studies on surgical mortality after laparoscopic PEH, the study authors determined the mean incidence to be 1.38%. Five studies were reviewed to determine the rate of progression from asymptomatic PEH to acute change requiring emergency surgery. The mean rate was 1.16% per year. Using these numbers, the computer program calculated that elective laparoscopic PEH repair in patients age 65 or older resulted in a reduction in quality-adjusted life years by 0.13. As the patients age increased, the quality-adjusted life continued to decline, obviating any surgical benefit. Restated, if laparoscopic PEH repair were instituted on all asymptomatic patients older than age 65, only 1 in 5 would benefit. In patients age 85 only 1 in 10 would benefit. Although strictly a computer model, this study adds support to the conservative treatment approach toward asymptomatic PEH. At the University of Washington, we have adopted a policy of nonoperative management in asymptomatic PEH patients who have associated high operative risks or advanced age.

Approach

Since its introduction, laparoscopy has gained rapid acceptance as the preferred method of PEH repair. Table 1 displays outcomes from laparoscopic PEH repair trials. Multiple studies validate the improvement in postoperative pain, recovery, and length of stay. Additionally, operative morbidity and mortality is lower with this approach. Recurrence rates have been alarmingly high, however, especially in early trials. It is difficult to compare open and laparoscopic results, because older open data do not routinely include esophagrams to identify asymptomatic recurrences. Most recurrence in the laparoscopic trials are small, asymptomatic, and only found with routine postoperative esophagrams. The significance of asymptomatic recurrence is unknown. Many authors advocate conservative management of these patients, because their natural history or incidence of progressing to complication is unknown.

Hashemi and colleagues [8] published one of the few comparisons of laparoscopic and open PEH repair. Recurrent hernia was documented by esophagram in 42% of the laparoscopic group and 15% of the open group ($P < 0.001$), though this was not a randomized study and significant selection bias may exist. Both groups included a small number of patients (21 and 20, respectively), and included the earliest experience of laparoscopic repairs in a mature esophageal surgical practice. Furthermore, the 42% recurrence rate in the laparoscopic group is the highest reported in the literature, with more recent studies citing a 5.5% to 22% recurrence rate (see Table 1) [9–13].

Table 1
Review of recent major published outcomes of laparoscopic PEH repair

Study	n	Follow-up (months)	Coversion rate (%)	Morbidity (%)	Mortality (%)	Operative time (min)	Length of stay (days)	Anatomic recurrence[a] (%)	Symptomatic recurrence (%)	Reoperative rate for recurrence (%)
Gantert 1999 [55]	55	11c	9.0	14.4	1.8	219b	2.4b	NR	5.4	4.0
Hashemi 2000 [8]	27	17c	7.4	11.0	0	184b	3.0c	42	NR	NR
Luketich 2000 [32]	100	12c	3.0	28.0	1.0	220c	2.0c	NR	NR	1.0
Wiechmann 2001 [10]	54	13c	10.0	NR	1.8	202b	NR	5.5	5.5	5.5
Khaitan 2002 [59]	25	25b	19.0	16.0	0	268b	2.9b	40	12	4.0
Mattar 2002 [56]	136	40b	2.2	10.2	2.2	218b	2.0c	33	4.4	2.0
Pierre 2002 [12]	200	18c	1.5	28.0	0.5	198c	3.0c	NR	NR	2.5
Diaz 2003 [11]	116	30b	2.5	4.3	1.7	162c	2.0c	22	11	2.6
Targarona 2004 [13]	37	24c	0	11.0	2.1	196b	4.0b	20	21	NR

Abbreviation: NR, not reported.
[a] Anatomic recurrence defined as recurrence identified by contrast radiography.
[b] Mean.
[c] Median.

Two studies have examined the quality of life after laparoscopic PEH repair. Using the Short Form 36 standard questionnaire, Velanovich and Karmy-Jones [14] showed that patients treated with laparoscopic PEH repair reported better quality of life (QOL) scores when compared with the open group. Targarona et al [13] assessed patients after laparoscopic PEH repair and reported postoperative QOL scores. Compared with a cohort of similar aged healthy patients, QOL scores were not statistically different. These studies attest to the improved QOL achieved via laparoscopic repair.

Operative techniques

Three fundamental steps are involved in PEH repair: (1) tension-free reduction of the esophagus and stomach into the abdomen with excision of the hernia sac; (2) reapproximation of the hiatus; and (3) subdiaphragmatic anchoring of the stomach, with many advocating the addition of an antireflux procedure.

Short esophagus

The first description of short esophagus was made by Lortat-Jacob in 1957 [15]. Since that time, the concept of a foreshortened esophagus has been established in the literature. Much debate has arisen regarding the incidence, importance, and treatment of short esophagus in patients who have PEH, however. Herbella and colleagues [16] performed a literature review of all antireflux surgical reports from 1998 to 2000, in an attempt to deduce the incidence of short esophagus. Although no common definition exists for short esophagus, after reviewing 94 papers with a total of 17,288 patients, they found the overall incidence to be 1.53%. The greatest risk factor associated with short esophagus was PEH. Of patients who have PEH, the incidence of short esophagus was 11.87%, more than 10 times greater than the overall incidence. The authors acknowledge that, as with all meta-analysis, significant biases exist, and that this likely does not represent the true incidence of short esophagus in patients who have PEH. They argue, however, that short esophagus truly exists, and that patients who have PEH are at increased risk.

The pathophysiology thought to be responsible for development of short esophagus in patients who have PEH is acid reflux or anatomic changes associated with herniation. Repeated exposure of the esophagus to reflux can lead to chronic inflammation and progressive damage to collagen elements. The resulting loss of esophageal elasticity can lead to fibrosis and contracture, resulting in short esophagus [17–19]. Anatomically, short esophagus may result when the esophagus accordions upon itself as stomach herniates into the chest. Subsequent formation of adhesions in the mediastinum results in varying degrees of difficulty obtaining esophageal length [18,19]. This has also been termed an apparent short esophagus, because mediastinal mobilization typically results in sufficient esophageal length. Regardless of the etiology of short esophagus, if not corrected, upward tension after repair of a PEH can result in increased recurrence [20].

Preoperative predictors of short esophagus have been sought to no avail in patients who have PEH. Preoperative tests do not reliably determine the need for an esophageal lengthening procedure. Gastal and associates [21] reported on 236 patients undergoing antireflux surgery. Of those patients, 37 (16%) had short esophagus and required a lengthening procedure. Although 18 (49%) patients had hiatal hernias ≥5 cm, this did not reach statistical significance ($P = 0.45$). Likewise, Awad and colleagues [22] found hiatal hernia size ≥5 cm did not accurately predict the need for an esophageal lengthening procedure. Ultimately, the diagnosis of short esophagus is made in the operating room after all attempts of achieving 2.5 cm of intra-abdominal esophageal length and a tension-free PEH repair have failed.

Esophageal mobilization

It is the authors' institutional experience that adequate dissection and mobilization of the mediastinal esophagus results in very few true, nonreducible short esophagi. With aggressive mobilization of the mediastinal esophagus via the laparoscopic approach, enough length is typically achieved to bring the gastroesophageal junction at least 2.5 cm below the hiatus. In the authors' cumulative experience, it is a rare occurrence when sufficient intra-abdominal esophagus cannot be achieved and a Collis gastroplasty is necessary. In support of this, Madan et al [23] recently published their series of 628 patients undergoing fundoplication. Over half of these patients (351) had a concomitant hiatal hernia, 11% (72) with a greater than 8-cm defect. Using laparoscopic mediastinal esophageal dissection, no patients required an esophageal lengthening procedure. All patients were evaluated for recurrence with an esophagram within the first year after surgery. With a mean follow-up of 4.3 years, they reported a failure rate of 2.6% (1.3% crural disruption, 0.5% slipped fundoplication, and 0.8% recurrence of reflux with and intact intra-abdominal wrap and crural closure). Similarly, O'Rourke et al [24] reported on their success with extended laparoscopic esophageal mobilization in an effort to avoid Collis gastroplasty. Circumferential blunt and harmonic scalpel dissection of the esophagus was performed, with care to preserve the main branches of the vagus nerve. On average, esophageal dissection was extended 7 to 10 cm into the mediastinum. In their retrospective study, 205 patients underwent laparoscopic Nissen fundoplication, 25 (12%) with Type II PEH. To obtain adequate esophageal length, extensive mobilization was required in 23 (92%) of patients who have PEH. On multivariate analysis, both the presence of a PEH on preoperative esophagram or hiatal hernia ≥5 cm were predictive of need to perform extensive mobilization ($P < 0.01$, $P < 0.001$ respectively). With an admitted short median follow-up of 8 months, only

1 patient had failure of the PEH repair. This study's 94% success rate is equivalent to those of reports with thoracotomy for extensive esophageal mobilization, with the significant advantage of avoiding painful thoracotomy and associated complications (reported as high as 42%) [19]. Extensive laparoscopic esophageal mobilization can provide sufficient esophageal length for repair of PEH while avoiding the disadvantages of both open surgery and Collis gastroplasty.

Collis gastroplasty

After all efforts to obtain adequate esophageal length have failed, a Collis gastroplasty may become necessary. The outcomes of this procedure are quite variable; thus the threshold for performing it differs among surgeons. Since first described by Orringer and Sloan in 1978 [25], the Collis-Nissen procedure has become the gastroplasty procedure of choice. Stirling and Orringer [26] published long-term follow-up of patients undergoing open Collis-Nissen gastroplasty. The mean follow-up was 43.8 months and included a high percentage of patients who have sliding hiatal hernia or PEH (72% and 17%, respectively). Reflux was eliminated or rated as mild in 86% of patients. Twenty-four hour pH monitoring demonstrated good reflux control in 91%. The overall mortality rate was 1.1%, with a complication rate of 8%. Complications included post-thoracotomy pain (8%), esophageal or gastroplasty leak (1.7%), and crural repair dehiscence (<1%). Ten percent of patients required reoperation for persistent reflux or dysphagia.

Others report inferior results. Swanstrom and associates [27] described the technique of laparoscopic Collis-Nissen, and reported their results in 15 consecutive patients. Follow-up at 14 months revealed symptomatic heartburn in 2 patients (14%), abnormal 24-hour pH study in 7 (50%, mean DeMeester score 100), persistent esophagitis in 5 (33%), and new onset distal esophageal aperistalsis in 6 (40%) [28]. Similarly, Lin and colleagues [29] showed that after mean follow-up of 30 months, 80% of patients undergoing a Collis gastroplasty have esophagitis on endoscopy and pathologic acid exposure on pH testing. Of 58 patients available for follow-up, 2 patients developed Barrett's esophagus. Certainly the creation of neoesophagus leaves acid-producing cells proximal to the intact fundoplication, potentially leading to pooling of acid in the neo- and distal esophagus, inflammation, and possible progression to Barrett's. For this reason, patients treated with a Collis gastroplasty should undergo routine endoscopic surveillance and pharmacologic acid suppression.

Hernia sac excision

Multiple studies have demonstrated the importance of complete sac excision after reduction of viscera into the abdomen [9,30–32]. Edye et al [30] showed hernia sac resection is a necessary step to prevent recurrence. Patients treated without sac excision had a recurrence rate of 20%, versus zero recurrence in the sac resection group ($P < 0.05$). The importance of this step is threefold. First, the stretched hernia sac produces upward traction on the stomach and esophagus. To prevent cephalad tension, the sac must be excised. Second, improved visualization of the gastroesophageal junction is achieved with sac removal. Finally, when reducing the stomach, the sac is used as a lever and is grasped instead of the stomach, thus preventing gastric wall injury or perforation.

Reapproximation of the hiatus

Closure of the hiatus is an essential step in PEH repair. Assessing why fundoplications fail, Horgan and coauthors [33] found that a majority (59%) can be attributed to loss of integrity of the crural closure and herniation of the gastroesophageal junction or stomach into the thorax. Soper and Dunnegan [34] examined 290 patients undergoing laparoscopic antireflux surgery and found a 7% incidence of postoperative intrathoracic migration of the wrap. Early in this series, patient were not treated with routine crural closure, resulting in a 19% failure rate. Later, all patients underwent posterior crural reapproximation and the rate dropped to 4% ($P < 0.05$).

Factors that need to be accessed before PEH repair include the stoutness of the crura and space between them. If the crura are not of sufficient girth, adequate suture purchase is not possible. Likewise, if the gap between crura is excessive, undue tension is placed on the sutures. Buttressing the hiatal closure, typically with a mesh onlay, is advocated by some authors [35–37]. Material such as polypropylene, polytetrafluoroethylene (PTFE), and porcine small-intestine submucosa are all used with differing success (Table 2). Although tension-free hiatal closure using prosthetic material intuitively seems superior to simple closure, reports of prosthetic erosion, stricture, and ulceration have tempered excitement [38]. The authors' experience is that reinforcement of the hiatus with prosthetic material is seldom necessary, and is used selectively in cases of significant tension.

Subdiaphragmatic anchoring of the stomach

Various techniques (fundoplication, gastrostomy, and anterior gastro-pexy) have been used to keep the stomach intra-abdominal and prevent recurrent PEH. In the early experience with open PEH repair, gastropexy was the most popular anchoring method; however, long-term follow-up of these patients found a high incidence of recurrence [11,39,40]. Ellis et al [40] reported on a series of 51 patients undergoing open PEH repair, and found Stamm gastrostomy superior to gastropexy in anchoring the stomach intra-abdominally and preventing recurrence. With the advent of laparoscopic PEH repair, this controversy has resurged. Ponsky and coworkers [41] recently published a prospective study in which 28 patients who had Type III PEH underwent laparoscopic repair with anterior gastropexy. No recurrence was reported with a mean follow-up of 21 months and all

Table 2
Review of clinical trials involving prosthetic reinforcement of PEH repair

Study	n	Follow-up (months)	Material	Placement	LOS (days)	Operaitve Time (min)	Morbidity (%)	Mortality (%)	Recurrence (%)	Complication due to prosthetic
Carlson 1998 [38][a]	44	51.6[b]	Polypropylene	Onlay/ keyhole	11[c]	NR	48	2	0	2% mesh erosion
Champion 2003 [36]	52	25.0[b]	Polypropylene	Onlay over crura	NR	101[b]	0	0	1.9	0
Hui 2001 [60]	12	37.0[b]	Polypropylene and PTFE	Onlay over crura	6[b]	226[b]	25	0	8.3	0
Frantzides 2002 [37]	36	39.6[b]	PTFE	Onlay/ keyhole	2[b]	156[b]	5.5	0	0	0
Oelschlager 2003 [35]	9	8.0[c]	SIS	Onlay/ Keyhole and U-shape	NR	NR	11	11	11	0

Abbreviations: LOS, length of stay; PTFE, polytetrafluoroethylene; SIS, porcine small intestine submucosa.
[a] All performed in an open fashion.
[b] Mean.
[c] Median.

patients underwent postoperative esophagrams. Likewise, gastrostomies have resurged as an anchoring method when performing laparoscopic repair. Kercher and colleagues [42] reported on successful laparoscopic-assisted PEH reduction and fixation with two percutaneous endoscopic gastrostomy tubes. They advocate this as a less invasive method of treating symptomatic PEH in high-risk surgical patients. With the lack of a definitive prospective randomized trial validating the use of gastropexy or gastrostomy, controversy regarding their utility is likely to remain.

Fundoplication

The incorporation of the Nissen fundoplication with PEH repair has gained popularity since Polk and Zeppa's successful report of 56 patients in 1969 [43]. The rationale for fundoplication is threefold. First, 30% to 85% of PEH patients report symptomatic reflux preoperatively [10,41,44,45]. If invasive 24-hour pH and esophageal manometry testing is performed on these patients, abnormal reflux and hypotensive lower esophageal sphincter pressures can be demonstrated in 60% to 100% of patients [46,47]. Second, the extensive dissection at the hiatus necessary to reduce the PEH and obtain sufficient intra-abdominal esophageal length results in a high (18%–65%) rate of postoperative reflux [48–50]. The hiatal dissection is thought to ablate the anatomic support responsible for gastroesophageal competence [6,46,51,52]. Finally, fundoplication anchors the stomach in the subdiaphragmatic position, potentially reducing recurrence [53].

Critics of routine fundoplication cite associated increases in operative time as well as the potential for postoperative dysphagia. Certainly, shorter operative time is a consideration in the typical elderly PEH patient who has multiple comorbidities; however, in experienced hands, fundoplication can be completed with minimal prolongation of operative time. As for dysphagia, the authors have experienced very little dysphagia after routine fundoplication in these patients [54]. Similar success with fundoplication has been reported elsewhere [10,13,32,55,56].

Multiple authors have shown routine fundoplication with PEH repair as an effective method to prevent postoperative reflux and affix the stomach intra-abdominally [10,41,53,54,57,58]. The type of fundoplication (Dor, Toupet, Nissen) remains surgeon preference. At the University of Washington, we perform Nissen fundoplications on all PEH patients who demonstrate normal preoperative esophageal motility.

Summary

As studies further define the natural history of PEH, mandatory surgical repair of asymptomatic patients is becoming more controversial. With the advent of minimally invasive techniques, morbidity and mortality associated with operative repair have declined; however, a high incidence of asymptomatic anatomic recurrence has been demonstrated with routine postoperative radiologic studies. The significance of this remains unknown. Are these patients at the same risk for strangulation and volvulus as they were before repair? Likely not, but no long-term studies have defined the risk.

At the University of Washington, we believe that the laparoscopic approach to PEH is the preferred method of repair. Its advantages include a reduction in morbidity and mortality, postoperative pain, length of stay, and convalescence. These are important factors in the typical debilitated elderly patient presenting with PEH. Fundamentals of the operation include: (1) tension free reduction of the stomach and esophagus with hernia sac resection, (2) crural closure, and (3) subdiaphragmatic anchoring of the stomach with an antireflux procedure. When these are performed, excellent symptomatic relief and prolonged anatomic repair can be achieved.

References

[1] Perdikis GH. Laparoscopic paraesophageal hernia repair. In: Eubanks WS SL, Soper NJ, editor. Mastery of endoscopic and laparoscopic surgery. Philadelphia: Lippincott Williams & Wilkins; 2000. p. 165–73.

[2] Hill LD. Incarcerated paraesophageal hernia. A surgical emergency. Am J Surg 1973;126(2): 286–91.

[3] Skinner DB, Belsey RH. Surgical management of esophageal reflux and hiatus hernia. Long-term results with 1030 patients. J Thorac Cardiovasc Surg 1967;53(1):33–54.

[4] Floch NR. Paraesophageal hernias: current concepts. J Clin Gastroenterol 1999;29(1):6–7.

[5] Hashemi M, Sillin LF, Peters JH. Current concepts in the management of paraesophageal hiatal hernia. J Clin Gastroenterol 1999;29(1):8–13.

[6] Allen MS, Trastek VF, Deschamps C, et al. Intrathoracic stomach. Presentation and results of operation. J Thorac Cardiovasc Surg 1993;105(2):253–8 [discussion: 258–9].

[7] Stylopoulos N, Gazelle GS, Rattner DW. Paraesophageal hernias: operation or observation? Ann Surg 2002;236(4):492–500 [discussion: 492–500].

[8] Hashemi M, Peters JH, DeMeester TR, et al. Laparoscopic repair of large Type III hiatal hernia: objective followup reveals high recurrence rate. J Am Coll Surg 2000;190(5):553–60 [discussion: 553–60].

[9] Leeder PC, Smith G, Dehn TC. Laparoscopic management of large paraesophageal hiatal hernia. Surg Endosc 2003;17(9):1372–5.

[10] Wiechmann RJ, Ferguson MK, Naunheim KS, et al. Laparoscopic management of giant paraesophageal herniation. Ann Thorac Surg 2001;71(4):1080–6 [discussion: 1086–7].

[11] Diaz S, Brunt LM, Klingensmith ME, et al. Laparoscopic paraesophageal hernia repair, a challenging operation: medium-term outcome of 116 patients. J Gastrointest Surg 2003; 7(1):59–66 [discussion: 59–66].

[12] Pierre AF, Luketich JD, Fernando HC, et al. Results of laparoscopic repair of giant paraesophageal hernias: 200 consecutive patients. Ann Thorac Surg 2002;74(6):1909–15 [discussion: 1909–15].

[13] Targarona EM, Novell J, Vela S, et al. Mid term analysis of safety and quality of life after the laparoscopic repair of paraesophageal hiatal hernia. Surg Endosc 2004;18(7):1045–50.

[14] Velanovich V, Karmy-Jones R. Surgical management of paraesophageal hernias: outcome and quality of life analysis. Dig Surg 2001;18(6):432–7 [discussion: 437–8].

[15] Lorstat-Jacob JL. L'endo-brachyesophage. Ann Chir 1957;11:1247.

[16] Herbella FA, Del Grande JC, Colleoni R. Short esophagus: literature incidence. Dis Esophagus 2002;15(2):125–31.

[17] Gozzetti G, Pilotti V, Spangaro M, et al. Pathophysiology and natural history of acquired short esophagus. Surgery 1987;102(3):507–14.

[18] Awad ZT, Filipi CJ. The short esophagus: pathogenesis, diagnosis, and current surgical options. Arch Surg 2001;136(1):113–4.

[19] Altorki NK, Yankelevitz D, Skinner DB. Massive hiatal hernias: the anatomic basis of repair. J Thorac Cardiovasc Surg 1998;115(4):828–35.

[20] Horvath KD, Swanstrom LL, Jobe BA. The short esophagus: pathophysiology, incidence, presentation, and treatment in the era of laparoscopic antireflux surgery. Ann Surg 2000; 232(5):630–40.

[21] Gastal OL, Hagen JA, Peters JH, et al. Short esophagus: analysis of predictors and clinical implications. Arch Surg 1999;134(6):633–6 [discussion: 637–8].

[22] Awad ZT, Mittal SK, Roth TA, et al. Esophageal shortening during the era of laparoscopic surgery. World J Surg 2001;25(5):558–61.

[23] Madan AK, Frantzides CT, Patsavas KL. The myth of the short esophagus. Surg Endosc 2004;18(1):31–4.

[24] O'Rourke RW, Khajanchee YS, Urbach DR, et al. Extended transmediastinal dissection: an alternative to gastroplasty for short esophagus. Arch Surg 2003;138(7):735–40.

[25] Orringer MB, Sloan H. Combined Collis-Nissen reconstruction of the esophagogastric junction. Ann Thorac Surg 1978;25(1):16–21.

[26] Stirling MC, Orringer MB. Continued assessment of the combined Collis-Nissen operation. Ann Thorac Surg 1989;47(2):224–30.

[27] Swanstrom LL, Marcus DR, Galloway GQ. Laparoscopic Collis gastroplasty is the treatment of choice for the shortened esophagus. Am J Surg 1996;171(5):477–81.

[28] Jobe BA, Horvath KD, Swanstrom LL. Postoperative function following laparoscopic Collis gastroplasty for shortened esophagus. Arch Surg 1998;133(8):867–74.

[29] Lin E, Swafford V, Chadalavada R, et al. Disparity between symptomatic and physiologic outcomes following esophageal lengthening procedures for antireflux surgery. J Gastrointest Surg 2004;8(1):31–9 [discussion: 31–8].

[30] Edye M, Salky B, Posner A, Fierer A. Sac excision is essential to adequate laparoscopic repair of paraesophageal hernia. Surg Endosc 1998;12(10):1259–63.

[31] Geha AS, Massad MG, Snow NJ, et al. A 32-year experience in 100 patients with giant paraesophageal hernia: the case for abdominal approach and selective antireflux repair. Surgery 2000;128(4):623–30.

[32] Luketich JD, Raja S, Fernando HC, et al. Laparoscopic repair of giant paraesophageal hernia: 100 consecutive cases. Ann Surg 2000;232(4):608–18.

[33] Horgan S, Pohl D, Bogetti D, et al. Failed antireflux surgery: what have we learned from reoperations? Arch Surg 1999;134(8):809–15 [discussion: 809–15].

[34] Soper NJ, Dunnegan D. Anatomic fundoplication failure after laparoscopic antireflux surgery. Ann Surg 1999;229(5):669–76 [discussion: 669–76].

[35] Oelschlager BK, Barreca M, Chang L, et al. The use of small intestine submucosa in the repair of paraesophageal hernias: initial observations of a new technique. Am J Surg 2003; 186(1):4–8.

[36] Champion JK, Rock D. Laparoscopic mesh cruroplasty for large paraesophageal hernias. Surg Endosc 2003;17(4):551–3.

[37] Frantzides CT, Madan AK, Carlson MA, et al. A prospective, randomized trial of laparoscopic polytetrafluoroethylene (PTFE) patch repair vs simple cruroplasty for large hiatal hernia. Arch Surg 2002;137(6):649–52.

[38] Carlson MA, Condon RE, Ludwig KA, et al. Management of intrathoracic stomach with polypropylene mesh prosthesis reinforced transabdominal hiatus hernia repair. J Am Coll Surg 1998;187(3):227–30.

[39] Braslow L. Transverse gastropexy vs Stamm gastrostomy in hiatal hernia. Arch Surg 1987; 122(7):851.

[40] Ellis FH Jr, Crozier RE, Shea JA. Paraesophageal hiatus hernia. Arch Surg 1986;121(4): 416–20.

[41] Ponsky J, Rosen M, Fanning A, et al. Anterior gastropexy may reduce the recurrence rate after laparoscopic paraesophageal hernia repair. Surg Endosc 2003;17(7):1029–35.

[42] Kercher KW, Matthews BD, Ponsky JL, et al. Minimally invasive management of paraesophageal herniation in the high-risk surgical patient. Am J Surg 2001;182(5):510–4.

[43] Polk HC Jr, Zeppa R. Fundoplication for complicated hiatal hernia. Rationale and results. Ann Thorac Surg 1969;7(3):202–11.

[44] Fuller CB, Hagen JA, DeMeester TR, et al. The role of fundoplication in the treatment of Type II paraesophageal hernia. J Thorac Cardiovasc Surg 1996;111(3):655–61.

[45] Williamson WA, Ellis FH Jr, Streitz JM Jr, et al. Paraesophageal hiatal hernia: is an antireflux procedure necessary? Ann Thorac Surg 1993;56(3):447–51 [discussion: 447–51].

[46] Walther B, DeMeester TR, Lafontaine E, et al. Effect of paraesophageal hernia on sphincter function and its implication on surgical therapy. Am J Surg 1984;147(1):111–6.

[47] Wo JM, Branum GD, Hunter JG, et al. Clinical features of Type III (mixed) paraesophageal hernia. Am J Gastroenterol 1996;91(5):914–6.

[48] Hill LD, Tobias JA. Paraesophageal hernia. Arch Surg 1968;96(5):735–44.

[49] Pearson FG, Cooper JD, Ilves R, et al. Massive hiatal hernia with incarceration: a report of 53 cases. Ann Thorac Surg 1983;35(1):45–51.

[50] Treacy PJ, Jamieson GG. An approach to the management of para-oesophageal hiatus hernias. Aust N Z J Surg 1987;57(11):813–7.

[51] Ellis FH Jr. Diaphragmatic hiatal hernias. Recognizing and treating the major types. Postgrad Med 1990;88(1):113–4; 117–20; 113–20.

[52] Wu JS, Dunnegan DL, Soper NJ. Clinical and radiologic assessment of laparoscopic paraesophageal hernia repair. Surg Endosc 1999;13(5):497–502.

[53] Casabella F, Sinanan M, Horgan S, et al. Systematic use of gastric fundoplication in laparoscopic repair of paraesophageal hernias. Am J Surg 1996;171(5):485–9.

[54] Horgan S, Eubanks TR, Jacobsen G, et al. Repair of paraesophageal hernias. Am J Surg 1999;177(5):354–8.

[55] Gantert WA, Patti MG, Arcerito M, et al. Laparoscopic repair of paraesophageal hiatal hernias. J Am Coll Surg 1998;186(4):428–32 [discussion: 428–32].

[56] Mattar SG, Bowers SP, Galloway KD, et al. Long-term outcome of laparoscopic repair of paraesophageal hernia. Surg Endosc 2002;16(5):745–9.

[57] Athanasakis H, Tzortzinis A, Tsiaoussis J, et al. Laparoscopic repair of paraesophageal hernia. Endoscopy 2001;33(7):590–4.

[58] Oelschlager BK, Pellegrini CA. Paraesophageal hernias: open, laparoscopic, or thoracic repair? Chest Surg Clin N Am 2001;11(3):589–603.

[59] Khaitan L, Houston H, Sharp K, et al. Laparoscopic paraesophageal hernia repair has an acceptable recurrence rate. Am Surg 2002;68(6):546–51 [discussion: 546–51].

[60] Hui TT, Thoman DS, Spyrou M, et al. Mesh crural repair of large paraesophageal hiatal hernias. Am Surg 2001;67(12):1170–4.

ELSEVIER
SAUNDERS

SURGICAL
CLINICS OF
NORTH AMERICA

Surg Clin N Am 85 (2005) 119–127

Laparoscopic gastric bypass for refractory morbid obesity

Conrad H. Simpfendorfer, MD, Samuel Szomstein, MD, Raul Rosenthal, MD, FACS*

Department of General and Vascular Surgery, Cleveland Clinic Florida, 2950 Cleveland Clinic Boulevard, Weston, FL 33331, USA

The problem of obesity in the United States has reached epidemic proportions [1,2]. The National Health and Nutrition Examination Survey recently reported that 34.9% of US adults are overweight or obese [1,3,4]. The increasing prevalence of obesity and its associated morbidity have by some accounts led to obesity surpassing tobacco abuse as the number one contributor to death and disease [5]. The mortality rates in the morbidly obese are 12 times higher in men aged 25 to 34 years and six times higher in men aged 35 to 44 years compared with nonobese men of the same age ranges [6]. Comorbid conditions such as hypertension, dyslipidemia, coronary heart disease, diabetes mellitus, gallbladder disease, arthritis, respiratory disease, gout, and many types of cancer are also increased in obese adults [1,7,8].

Because of the failures of conservative treatment options, such as low-calorie diets, exercise programs, and behavior modifications, as well as current medical treatments, several surgical procedures have been developed that have proven to be effective in achieving long-term weight reduction [9,10]. As a result, the number of patients undergoing bariatric surgery has increased dramatically in recent years. With an estimated 80,000 bariatric surgeries performed in 2002 [9,11] and 103,000 in 2003 [12].

The number of practicing surgeons who are members of the American Society for Bariatric Surgery (ASBS) has increased from 258 in 1998 to 1070 in 2003. Two major trends in the last decade were recognized in a survey of members of the ASBS in 1999 [13]. First, Roux-en-Y gastric bypass (RYGBP) was the most commonly performed bariatric operation, with a frequency of 70%. Second, laparoscopic procedures were emerging, with

* Corresponding author.
E-mail address: rosentr@ccf.org (R. Rosenthal).

0039-6109/05/$ - see front matter © 2005 Elsevier Inc. All rights reserved.
doi:10.1016/j.suc.2004.10.001   surgical.theclinics.com

a frequency of only 3% in 1999. In 2003, about 56% of all bariatric operations were performed laparoscopically, according to the ASBS.

History

Mason and Ito [14] introduced the concept of gastric bypass in the treatment of morbid obesity in 1967. Over the ensuing decade, Mason and his colleagues at the University of Iowa [15] refined the concept of gastric restriction. They emphasized the measurement limitations for both the volume of the upper gastric pouch and the diameter of the gastro-jejunostomy. Modifications to Mason's gastric bypass, using a divided stomach, were followed by Alden's 1977 series of successfully partitioned stomachs using intestinal staplers [16]. In the same year, Griffen et al [17] published the first series using an RYGBP rather than a loop gastro-jejunostomy. During the 1980s, the field of bariatric surgery underwent many transitions, with the abandonment of the jejunoileal bypass and the wide acceptance and application of gastric restriction by stapled gastro-plasty. Surgeons who continued to perform gastric bypass as the procedure of choice primarily used a RYGBP technique over the loop approach. Significant evidence exists documenting both the short-term and long-term results of open RYGBP. Selected series demonstrate long-term weight loss at 5 to 15 years to be 49% to 62% of excess body weight [13].

In 1994, Wittgrove and Clark [18] were the first to describe laparoscopic Roux-en-Y gastric bypass (LRYGBP). Their technique involves creation of a 15- to 30-mL gastric pouch isolated from the distal stomach, a 21-mm stapled circular anastomosis, a 75-cm retrocolic retrogastric Roux-limb, and a stapled jejunojejunal anastomosis. With the introduction of less invasive techniques to bariatric surgery, a reduction in perioperative morbidity was found to be the major advantage, primarily related to cardiopulmonary and wound complications [13,19,20].

Laparoscopic gastric bypass

The gastric bypass operation is the most commonly performed operation for morbid obesity in the United States. The laparoscopic approach simulates the open procedure, and not surprisingly, LRYGBP has become the most prevalent laparoscopic bariatric procedure in the United States. Several reports have validated its safety, feasibility, and cost effectiveness, with decreased morbidity and comparable weight loss compared with the open technique [21–26]. The results of three prospective randomized studies comparing laparoscopic versus open RYGBP are shown in Table 1. Other advantages of the LRYGBP include reduced operative blood loss, less postoperative pain, lower pulmonary complications, a shorter hospital stay, a shorter return to normal activities, and a better quality of life

Table 1
Comparison of randomized laparoscopic versus open gastric bypass

Parameter	Lujan et al [24]		Nguyen et al [25]		Westling et al [26]	
Approach	Lap	Open	Lap	Open	Lap	Open
Number	53	51	79	76	30	21
Operative time (min)	186	202	225	195	235	100
Conversions (%)	8		2.5		23	
Early complications (%)	23	29	7.6	9.2	23	4.7
Late complications (%)	11	24	18.9	15.2	23	33
Mean LOS (d)	5.2	7.9	4	8.4	4	6

Abbreviations: Lap, laparoscopy; LOS, length of stay.

Adapted from Brolin RE. Laparoscopic versus open gastric bypass to treat morbid obesity. Ann Surg 2004;239:438–40; with permission.

[13,23,25,27–29]. Table 2 demonstrates a comparison of some of the larger cohort studies of LRYGBP.

Since the first description of the LRYGBP by Wittgrove and Clark [18] in 1994, multiple variations to the procedure have been introduced. Technical alternatives exist in the formation of the gastric pouch, creation of the gastrojejunal anastomosis, and the orientation and length of the alimentary limb. The gastrojejunostomy may be constructed by EEA circular stapler, GIA linear stapler, hand-sewn technique, or a combination of stapler and hand-sewn technique. Originally, the anvil of the EEA was introduced through the mouth and exited through the gastric pouch using a pull-wire technique. This procedure was later modified by de la Torre and Scott [30] in 1999, by introducing the anvil intra-abdominally, allowing greater precision of anvil placement, and avoiding esophageal injury. In 2000, Higa and

Table 2
Laparoscopic Roux-en-Y gastric bypass: outcomes

Reference	N	Female (%)	BMI	Mean OR time (min)	Conversions (%)	LOS (d)	Overall complications (%)	EWL (mo)
Higa et al [27]	1500	81	NA	NA	1.3	1.5	14.8	69% (12)
Kennedy et al (submitted for publication, 2004)	849	80	56	95	0.6	3.9	30.6	73% (12)
Wittgrove et al [28]	500	NA	NA	120	NA	2.6	12.6	73% (54)
DeMaria et al [29]	281	87	48	162[a]	2.8	4	23	70% (12)
Schauer et al [23]	275	81	48	247	1.1	2.6	30.3	77% (30)

Abbreviations: BMI, body mass index; EWL, estimated weight loss; LOS, length of stay; NA, not available; OR, operating room.

[a] Last 70 patients.

associates [22] described a technique for hand-sewn gastrojejunostomy in an attempt to reduce anastomotic leaks. Other alternatives in operative technique exist in the orientation and length of the Roux limb. The Roux limb may be positioned retro-colic versus ante-colic, and the gastro-jejunostomy constructed either retro-gastric versus ante-gastric. Shauer and coworkers [23] performed a retro-colic, retro-gastric Roux limb, with creation of the gastrojejunostomy using the linear stapler, whereas we and other groups [31] use an ante-colic, ante-gastric Roux limb and a linear stapler for the gastrojejunostomy. The length of the Roux limb may vary from 75 to 200 cm, according to the patient's body mass index (BMI), with institutions using different sets of criteria for alimentary limb lengths. Despite the lack of consensus regarding the specific technical aspects of LRYGBP, the hallmarks of the surgery remain universal with respect to formation of a small volume gastric pouch (15–30 mL), creation of a restrictive gastrojejunostomy, and construction of a malabsorptive limb of variable length.

Results

Although open RYGBP may be considered the gold standard, early results of LRYGBP compare favorably. In a randomized study of outcomes after laparoscopic and open RYGBP, Nguyen et al [25] presented a 155-patient series (79 laparoscopic, 76 open) with a 2-year follow-up (see Table 1). Both groups had similar initial excess weight loss (IEWL) at 1 year: 68% in the laparoscopic and 62% in the open group. The mean operative time for the laparoscopic (225 ± 40 minutes) was greater than for the open operation (195 ± 41 minutes). Not surprisingly, the relative complications included a lower incidence of wound infection (1.3%) and a lower incidence of incisional hernia (0.0%) in the laparoscopic group compared with those of the open group (10.5% and 6.6%, respectively). In addition, patients who had LRYGBP developed significantly less pulmonary impairment, with fewer patients developing segmental atelectasis requiring supplemental oxygen, than patients in the open group. Of interest, this study noted an increase in late anastomotic stricture rate in the LRYGBP (11.4%) as compared with the open RYGBP group (2.6%).

Schauer and Ikramuddin [13] presented a review of the published experience with LRYGBP. They noted that operating times ranged from 2 to 4 hours, and appeared to increase with increasing BMI, but decreased with experience; conversion rates were less than 5%. The mortality rate after LRYGBP ranged between 0% and 1.5%, comparable to that of open RYGBP. Both early (3.3%–15%), and late (2.2%–27%) complications were reasonably low, and the mean hospital stay was 2 to 3 days. Most series demonstrated a favorable IEWL of 65% to 80%, with a mean follow-up of 2 years. Furthermore, most authors reported that the majority of comorbid-ities, such as type 2 diabetes, sleep apnea, and hypertension, were improved or resolved with weight loss [32]. Kennedy et al (submitted for publication, 2004) presented similar results in 849 patients who underwent LRYGBP, with 844 (99.4%) of the procedures completed laparoscopically, and a mean operative time of 95 minutes (50–157 minutes) (see Table 2). The mean excess weight loss at 1 year was 73.4%, with no mortality and a major complication rate of 11.2% (Kennedy et al, submitted for publication, 2004). This included 53 patients (6.2%) who had anastomotic stricture, 21 patients (2.5%) with postoperative bleeding, 16 patients (1.8%) with anastomotic leak, and 2 patients (0.2%) with small-bowel obstruction.

Although cardiopulmonary and wound-related complications are much reduced after LRYGBP compared with open RYGBP, specific complications observed after LRYGBP include conversion to open operation, anastomotic intestinal leak, thromboembolism, hemorrhage, anastomotic stricture, marginal ulceration, hernia and bowel obstruction, cholelithiasis, and death. Table 3 lists the frequency of complications associated with laparoscopic gastric bypass.

Schauer et al [23] divided postoperative complications into early minor (27%), early major (3.3%), and late complications (47%). Major complications included two pulmonary embolisms, one which proved to be fatal, five leaks requiring surgical or percutaneous intervention, and three bowel obstructions requiring reoperation. Higa and associates [33], in a series of more than 1000 cases, reported the most common complications as stenosis at the gastrojejunostomy (4.9%), internal hernia (2.5%), marginal ulcer (1.4%), and staple line leaks (1%). Mortality in that series was reportedly 0.5%. Podnos and coauthors [34] recently reported complications in select series of LRYGBP. They reviewed 3464 cases, which were compared with a selected cohort of open gastric bypass, and demonstrated a decrease in wound-related complications and mortality in the laparoscopic group. They also noted an increased frequency of bowel obstruction, gastrointestinal tract hemorrhage, and stomal stenosis compared with the open series.

The incidences of both early and late bowel obstructions were found to be higher after LRYGBP compared with open gastric bypass, because of the lack of intra-abdominal adhesions and failure to close all potential defects that could lead to internal hernia. Potential defects include the transverse mesocolon defect in a retrocolic anastomosis, Petersen hernia (space between Roux-limb and transverse mesocolon), and the jejunojejunostomy mesenteric defect. Nguyen and coworkers retrospectively reviewed the charts of 9 (4%) of their initial 225 patients who developed postoperative bowel obstruction after LRYGBP [35]. Eight of the 9 patients required operative intervention, and 6 of the 8 were managed laparoscopically. Champion and Williams [36] reported an incidence of 13 (1.8%) patients who developed postoperative bowel obstruction requiring surgical intervention. The incidence of small bowel obstruction (SBO) was 4.5% (11/246) in the retrocolic group, and 0.43% (2/465) in the antecolic group, which

Table 3
Complications of laparoscopic gastric bypass in selected series

Reference	No. of patients	PE (%)	Leak (%)	Bowel obstruction (%)	GI bleeding (%)	Wound infection (%)	Stenosis (%)	Hernia (%)	Death (%)
Schauer et al [23]	275	2 (0.7)	12 (4.4)	3 (1.1)	3 (1.1)	24 (8.7)	13 (4.7)	2 (0.7)	1 (0.4)
Wittgrove et al [28]	500	NA	11 (2.2)	3 (0.6)	NA	28 (5.6)	8 (1.6)	0 (0)	0 (0)
Nguyen et al [25]	79	0 (0)	1 (1.3)	3 (3.8)	3 (3.8)	1 (1.3)	9 (11.4)	0 (0)	0 (0)
Higa et al [27]	1500	3 (0.2)	14 (0.9)	52 (3.5)	NA	2 (0.1)	73 (4.9)	4 (0.3)	3 (0.2)
Dresel et al [39]	100	0 (0)	3 (3)	5 (5)	3 (3)	2 (2)	3 (3)	1 (1)	0 (0)
DeMaria et al [29]	281	3 (1.1)	14 (4.9)	5 (1.8)	NA	3 (1.1)	18 (6.4)	5 (1.8)	0 (0)
Abdel-Galil et al [40]	90	NA	5 (5.5)	9 (10)	NA	NA	18 (20)	NA	0 (0)
Papasavas et al [41]	116	1 (0.8)	3 (2.6)	12 (10.3)	2 (1.7)	NA	4 (3.4)	NA	1 (0.8)
Oliak et al [42]	300	2 (0.6)	4 (1.3)	5 (1.7)	NA	20 (6.7)	6 (2.0)	NA	3 (1.0)
Gould et al [43]	223	NA	4 (1.8)	4 (1.8)	NA	17 (7.6)	12 (5.3)	2 (0.8)	0 (0)
Kennedy et al (Submitted for publication, 2004)	849	7 (0.8)	16 (1.8)	2 (0.2)	21 (2.5)	31 (3.6)	53 (6.2)	2 (0.2)	0 (0)
Total no.	4313	18/3500 (0.5)	87/4313 (2.0)	103/4313 (2.4)	32/1419 (2.3)	128/4107 (3.1)	217/4313 (5.0)	16/3807 (0.4)	8/4313 (0.18)

Abbreviations: GI, gastrointestinal; NA, not available; PE, pulmonary embolism.
Adapted from Podnos YD, Jimenez JC, Wilson SE, et al. Complications after laparoscopic gastric bypass. A review of 3464 cases. Arch Surg 2003;138:957–61; with permission.

was highly significant ($P = .006$). Performing an antecolic anastomosis eliminates the potential for obstruction at the transverse mesocolon defect.

Lomenzo et al [37] presented 40 patients who had gastrojejunal anastomotic strictures from 602 LRYGBP procedures (6.6%), with marginal ulcers noted in 4 of these patients. Treatment included a mean of two (range 1–4) dilations per patient. The time from original surgery to dilation of stricture ranged from 20 to 154 days (mean 52.7). The strictures ranged from 2 to 9 mm in size (mean 5.2) and dilations were performed using the through the scope (TTS) technique to a final diameter of 10 to 16.5 mm. None of these patients underwent surgical revision. Strictures at the gastrojejunostomy can be successfully and safely managed with endoscopic balloon dilation. Most patients present an average of 2.7 months after surgery, and often respond to one to two dilations [38]. Marginal ulcers were all managed with proton pump inhibitors and sucralfate.

Summary

Laparoscopic Roux-en-Y gastric bypass is fast becoming the gold standard for treatment of refractory morbid obesity in the United States. The minimally invasive approach accomplishes the same objectives as open RYGBP, but offers significant advantages in decreased perioperative morbidity, primarily with respect to the reduction in postoperative pain, lower rates of wound-related complications, decreased cardiopulmonary complications, and faster recovery. The accumulated early results of LRYGBP demonstrate that it is a technically feasible and safe operation, and that it has outcomes similar to those of open RYGBP.

The epidemic of obesity in the United States has led to an almost exponential annual increase in bariatric surgery. Fueled by the failure of diets, exercise, and medical therapy, and the publicity of new minimally invasive procedures, hospitals and surgeons are having a difficult time keeping up with the demand, and typically have long waiting lists for laparoscopic bariatric surgery. Given this demand, and the advanced surgical skills required in minimally invasive technique, particularly for LRYGBP, the ASBS has issued guidelines for granting bariatric-surgery privileges and for the establishment of "centers of excellence" programs. More systematic research on the basic mechanisms, physiology, and outcomes of bariatric surgery, particularly with respect to the new minimally invasive procedures, is necessary.

References

[1] Abir F, Bell R. Assessment and management of the obese patient. Crit Care Med 2004; 32(4 suppl):587–91.
[2] Modkad AH, Serdula M, Dietz W, et al. The continuing obesity epidemic in the United States. JAMA 2000;284:1650–1.

[3] Anonymous. Update: prevalence of overweight among children, adolescents and adults—United States 1988–1994. MMWR Morb Mortal Wkly Rep 1997;46:198–202.

[4] Kuczmarski RJ, Flegal KM, Campbell SM, et al. Increasing prevalence of overweight among US adults: The National Health and Nutrition Examination Surveys, 1960–1991. JAMA 1994;272:205–11.

[5] Sturm R. The effects of obesity, smoking, and drinking on medical problems and costs: obesity outranks both smoking and drinking in its deleterious effects on health costs. Health Aff 2002;21:245–53.

[6] Drenick EJ, Bale GS, Seltzer F, et al. Excessive mortality and causes of death in morbidly obese men. JAMA 1980;243:443–5.

[7] Health implications of obesity. National Institutes of Health Consensus Development Conference statement. Ann Intern Med 1985;103:147–51.

[8] Lew EA, Garfinkel L. Variations in mortality by weight among 750,000 men and women. J Chronic Dis 1979;32:563–76.

[9] Stocker DJ. Management of the bariatric surgery patient. Clin Endocrinol Metab 2003;32:2.

[10] Balsiger BM, Murr MM, Poggio JL, et al. Bariatric surgery. Surgery for weight control in patients with morbid obesity. Med Clin N Am 2000;84:477–89.

[11] Alt SJ. Bariatric surgery programs growing quickly nationwide. Health Care Strateg Manage 2001;19:7–23.

[12] Steinbrook R. Surgery for morbid obesity. N Engl J Med 2004;350(11):1075–9.

[13] Schauer PR, Ikramuddin S. Laparoscopic surgery for morbid obesity. Surg Clin N Am 2001; 81:1145–79.

[14] Mason EE, Ito CC. Gastric bypass in obesity. Surg Clin North Am 1967;47:1345–54.

[15] Mason EE, Printen KJ, Hartford CE, et al. Optimizing results of gastric bypass. Ann Surg 1975;182:405–14.

[16] Alden JF. Gastric and jejunoileal bypass: a comparison in the treatment of morbid obesity. Arch Surg 1997;112:799–804.

[17] Griffen WO Jr, Young L, Stevenson CC. A prospective comparison of gastric and jejunoileal bypass procedures for morbid obesity. Ann Surg 1977;186:500–9.

[18] Wittgrove AC, Clark GW. Laparoscopic gastric bypass, Roux-en-Y: preliminary report of five cases. Obes Surg 1994;4:353–7.

[19] Mason EE, Tang S, Renquist KE, et al. A decade of change in obesity surgery. Obes Surg 1997;7:189–97.

[20] Kellum JM, DeMaria EJ, Sugerman HJ. The surgical treatment of morbid obesity. Curr Probl Surg 1998;35:796–851.

[21] Livingston EH. Obesity and its surgical management. Am J Surg 2002;184:2.

[22] Higa KD, Boone KB, Ho T, et al. Laparoscopic Roux-en-Y gastric bypass for morbid obesity: technique and preliminary results of our first 400 patients. Arch Surg 2000;135: 1029–33.

[23] Schauer PR, Ikramuddin S, Gourash W, et al. Outcomes after laparoscopic Roux-en-Y gastric bypass for morbid obesity. Ann Surg 2000;232:515–29.

[24] Lujan JA, Frutos D, Hernandez Q, et al. Laparoscopic versus open gastric bypass in the treatment of morbid obesity. A randomized prospective study. Ann Surg 2004;239:433–7.

[25] Nguyen NT, Goldman C, Rosenquist J, et al. Laparoscopic versus open gastric bypass a randomized study of outcomes, quality-of-life, and costs. Ann Surg 2001;234:279–91.

[26] Westling A, Gustavson S. Laparoscopic vs. open Roux-en-Y gastric bypass: a prospective randomized trial. Obes Surg 2001;11:284–92.

[27] Higa KD, Ho T, Boone KB. Laparoscopic Roux-en-Y gastric bypass: technique and 3-year follow-up. J Laparoendosc Adv Surg Tech A 2001;11:377–82.

[28] Wittgrove AC, Clark WG. Laparoscopic gastric bypass, Roux-en-Y: 500 patients: technique and results, with 3–60 month follow-up. Obes Surg 2000;10:233–8.

[29] DeMaria EJ, Sugerman HJ, Kellum JM, et al. Results of 281 consecutive total laparoscopic Roux-en-Y gastric bypasses to treat morbid obesity. Ann Surg 2002;235:640–7.

[30] de la Torre RA, Scott JS. Laparoscopic Roux-en-Y gastric bypass a totally intra-abdominal approach—technique and preliminary report. Obes Surg 1999;9:492–8.
[31] Gagner M, Garcia-Ruiz A, Arca MJ, et al. Laparoscopic isolated gastric bypass for morbid obesity. Surg Endosc 1999;S19:6.
[32] Buchwald H. Overview of bariatric surgery. J Am Coll Surg 2002;194:3.
[33] Higa KD, Boone KB, et al. Complications of the laparoscopic Roux-en-Y gastric bypass: 1040 patients—what have we learned? Obes Surg 2000;10:509–13.
[34] Podnos YD, Jimenez JC, Wilson SE, et al. Complications after laparoscopic gastric bypass. A review of 3464 cases. Arch Surg 2003;138:957–61.
[35] Nguyen NT, Huerta S, Gelfand D, et al. Bowel obstruction after laparoscopic Roux-en-Y gastric bypass. Obes Surg 2004;14:190–6.
[36] Champion JK, Williams M. Small bowel obstruction and internal hernias after laparoscopic Roux-en-Y gastric bypass. Obes Surg 2003;13:596–600.
[37] Lomenzo E, Podkameni D, Kennedy C, et al. Gastrojejunal anastomotic stricture after laparoscopic Roux-en-Y gastric bypass. Presented at ASBS annual meeting. 2004.
[38] Ahmad J, Martin J, Ikramuddin S, et al. Endoscopic balloon dilation of the gastroenteric anastomotic stricture after laparoscopic gastric bypass. Endoscopy 2003;S35(9):725–8.
[39] Dresel A, Kuhn JA, Westmoreland MV, et al. Establishing a laparoscopic gastric bypass program. Am J Surg 2002;184:617–20.
[40] Abdel-Galil E, Sabry AA. Laparoscopic Roux-en-Y gastric bypass: evaluation of three different techniques. Obes Surg 2002;12:639–42.
[41] Papasavas PK, Hayetian FD, Caushaj BF, et al. Outcome analysis of laparoscopic Roux-en-Y gastric bypass for morbid obesity. Surg Endosc 2002;16:1653–7.
[42] Oliak D, Ballantyne GH, Davies RJ, et al. Short-term results of laparoscopic gastric bypass in patients with BMI ≥60. Obes Surg 2002;12:643–7.
[43] Gould JC, Needleman BJ, Ellison EC, et al. Evolution of minimally invasive bariatric surgery. Surgery 2002;132:565–72.

ELSEVIER
SAUNDERS

SURGICAL
CLINICS OF
NORTH AMERICA

Surg Clin N Am 85 (2005) 129–140

Laparoscopic adjustable gastric band

George A. Fielding, MBBS*, Christine J. Ren, MD

*Department of Surgery, New York University School of Medicine,
530 First Avenue, Suite 10 S, New York, NY 10016, USA*

Since Belachew [1] first performed the procedure in 1993, laparoscopic adjustable gastric banding (LAGB) has gained in popularity around the world as a first-choice surgical therapy for severely obese patients. LAGB is a purely restrictive operation that relies on decreased amount of intake as the mechanism for weight loss, and has less risk of malnutrition than with diversionary or bypass procedures. Adjustable gastric banding involves the surgical implantation of an inflatable silicone band around the uppermost part of the stomach, which is tightened in the office based on individual weight loss and appetite. Band tightening or adjustments are performed by percutaneously accessing a subcutaneous reservoir port that is connected to the band, and injecting fluid into the system. Band adjustments are required approximately five or six times in the first year and two or three times in the second year. Weight loss is gradual, averaging 1 to 2 lb per week during the first 2 years after surgery. The LAP-BAND System (Inamed Health, Santa Barbara, California) was the first device approved by the Federal Drug Administration (FDA) in 2001, and is presently the only adjustable gastric band available in the United States. Other versions exist internationally, one of which is in the approval process for use in the United States.

If one were asked to define a good minimally invasive bariatric procedure, there are some features that might be considered. Above all else, the procedure should be safe. There should be a reasonably quick operating room time and a low rate of conversion to open surgery. Hospital stay should be short, with minimal postoperative complications, especially related to wound and pulmonary difficulties, and patients should be able to return to work and normal activities as soon as they can. Ideally, there should be few long-term risks once the procedure is completed. The weight loss should be effective and lasting, and the symptomatic consequences of the procedure should be well tolerated by the majority of patients. If the

---

* Corresponding author.
E-mail address: george.fielding@med.nyu.edu (G.A. Fielding).

surgical.theclinics.com

patient cannot tolerate the procedure, it should be able to be converted to an alternate procedure, or completely reversed. Finally, it should be a procedure that is reproducible and teachable on a broad front to surgeons in training, and to any surgeon who is committed to the principles of bariatric surgery.

This article on LAGB for morbid obesity aims to address the issues raised in the preface to this edition concerning the effectiveness of the band as a minimally invasive procedure by assessing the above features as presented in recent literature.

Safety, conversion to open, and early complications

Virtually all published series of primary LAGB insertions have a conversion rate around 1%. This is usually due to hepatomegaly, or occasionally to adhesions. There are few comparative laparoscopic versus open data for LAGB. De Luca et al [2] compared 4-year results in 69 patients who underwent LAGB procedure by laparotomy or laparoscopy. Four open patients were reoperated to remove the band, and in 9 patients a ventral hernia appeared (5 patients repaired). In the laparoscopic cases there were 4 intraoperative gastric perforations, but all were repaired and the band placed at the same time (three conversions to open), causing an increased postoperative hospital stay. This is evidence of the learning curve. De Wit and colleagues [3] performed a prospective randomized trial comparing open and laparoscopic adjustable silicone gastric banding (LASGB) in 50 patients. The total number of readmissions (6 versus 15) and overall hospital stay in the first year (7.8 versus 11.8 days) were both lower after LASGB ($P < 0.05$). Weight and body mass index (BMI) were reduced significantly in both groups, but there was no difference between the groups. The laparoscopic procedure was associated with a shorter initial hospital stay and fewer readmissions during follow-up, and is therefore the preferred treatment.

There are some data comparing LAGB with other procedures that assess perioperative complications. Suter and associates [4] compared the early results of laparoscopic gastric banding and open vertical-banded gastro-plasty (VGB) in 197 patients. Mortality was similar, but the postoperative morbidity was higher in the VBG group (23.8% versus 8.0%, $P < 0.005$). The hospital stay was much shorter in the LAGB group; weight loss was less after 6 and 12 months, but was similar after 18 months in both groups.

LAGB is the safest bariatric operation available, with 0.05% mortality [5], 5% 30-day morbidity, and a delayed complication (gastric prolapse, erosion, port/tubing disconnection) rate of 12% [6–15]. O'Brien and Dixon [16] reviewed 1120 laparoscopic bands, and at 6 years have found no mortality. Weiner and coauthors [17] have 8-year data on 984 patients with zero mortality. A combined series [18] from Europe of 5827 patients has 0.2% mortality. Fielding and Duncombe [19] have 2110 bands at 7 years with 0.05% mortality. A combined Italian series [20] of 1265 patients with

BMI 44 has 0.5% mortality. The dominant theme of these longer-term follow-ups is that the laparoscopic band is very safe.

The Australian Safety and Efficacy Register of New Interventional Procedures-Surgical (ASERNIP-S), a government body whose role is to assess the safety and effectiveness of new procedures, evaluated the LAGB against open VBG and open Roux-en Y gastric bypass (RYGB) in terms of safety and efficacy. Their literature review (121 studies) [5] found LAGB to be safer than VBG and RYGB, and to be effective up to 4 years after surgery. Their conclusions were that in published literature, the laparoscopic band has mortality of 0.05%, compared with 0.5% for the gastric bypass. At 4 years, weight loss was the same, after an initial advantage to the RYGB. The median complication rate for LAGB was 11.3%, with very few studies reporting overall morbidity rates above 20% [5]. The frequency of complications is inversely related to surgeon experience with the procedure.

The ASERNIP-S review illustrated the relationship between the number of patients in the series and the incidence of complications. This underscores the learning curve associated with LAGB surgery, and may explain some of the early US center outcomes [21]. More importantly, the severity of complications after LAGB is significantly lower compared with gastrointestinal bypass operations.

When complications from LAGB, laparoscopic RYGB, and laparoscopic biliopancreatic diversion with duodenal switch (BPDDS) are compared according to severity (grade 1–4) and time of occurrence (early versus late), LAGB is the safest operation. A recent review of over 3000 patients with RYGB from one center over a 20+ years period of time [22] showed 1.5% mortality and 3.2% leak. Flum and Dellinger [23] recently reported a 1.9%, 30-day mortality in 3328 patients from Washington state undergoing RYGB. As ASERNIP-S recently reported, mortality was directly related to experience.

These data have recently been further supported by Laker et al [24], who compared risk of bad outcomes among LAGB, RYGB, and biliopancreatic diversion (BPD), all done laparoscopically, in a major teaching hospital in New York. In a study of 780 bariatric operations (480 LAGB, 235 RYGB, and 65 BPD) there was one late death after RYGB. Total complication rates were 9% for LAGB, 23% for RYGB, and 25% for BPD with or without duodenal switch (BPD ± DS). Complications resulting in organ resection, irreversible deficits, and death (Grades III and IV) occurred at rates of 0.2% for LAGB, 2% for RYGB, and 5% for BPD ± DS. The LAGB group had a statistically significant lower overall and severe complication rate compared with other groups ($P < 0.001$). After controlling for differences between the groups on age, admission BMI, gender, and race, LAGB patients had almost three and a half times lower likelihood of a complication compared with the RYGB group (OR = 3.4, 95% CI = 2.2–5.3, $P < 0.0001$). The odds ratio for developing complications after LAGB is 3.5 times lower than laparoscopic RYGB and laparoscopic malabsorptive operations.

Retrospective data from Biertho and colleagues [25] comparing LAGB to RYGB found a significantly lower postoperative major complication rate after LAGB (1.7%) compared with RYGB (4.2%). Fisher [26] recently showed that, in his hands, LAGB patients were discharged significantly quicker than after laparoscopic RYGB, and that LAGBs were able to resume normal activity at 7 days, compared with 18 days for laparoscopic RYGB ($P = 0.0002$). Dolan and coworkers [27] compared BPD and LAGB in 46 superobese (BMI >50) patients. Median excess weight loss at 24 months was 15% greater with BPD than with LAGB, but hospital stay and complication rates were also considerably greater with BPD. Rates of resolution of obstructive sleep apnea, hypertension, and diabetes mellitus following LAGB were similar to those of BPD. The researchers felt that the significant complication rate associated with BPD in superobesity outweighs any potential benefits of the extra weight loss gained over LAGB.

Complications

After Belechew [1] published his work in 1994, LAGB became popular in Europe, Australia, and Mexico. The technique has evolved considerably since then [28]. The first major change was evolution of the pars-flaccida approach to the esophagogastric angle, such that the band is placed out of the lesser sac. This has greatly reduced the incidence of gastric herniation through the band, the so-called "slip." The incidence of this complication has fallen from 12% in early series to 1% to 2% in current practice [18]. The second change was to leave the band uninflated at surgery, so that it remained loose while the gastro-gastric sutures healed. This has further reduced the chance of slip by eliminating vomiting in the early postoperative period. The adjustments to the band are done slowly and regularly, usually at 6- to 8-week intervals. This encourages regular attendance at follow-up and ensures a steady rate of weight loss. Finally, the adjustments are performed in the surgeon's office, based on the patients' hunger, rate of weight loss, and the volume of food they can eat. This has greatly simplified the adjustment schedule, and virtually eliminated the need for radiographs. These changes have led to high levels of patient tolerance of the laparoscopic band, and to sustainable weight loss.

Gastric prolapse, also known as band slippage, consists of herniation of the stomach up through the band cephalad, resulting in an enlarged gastric pouch, band malposition, and partial or complete gastric occlusion that typically presents as nocturnal vomiting. It occurs at a rate of 1.8% to 5% [29,30]. Band erosion occurs rarely (0%–7%), and appears to be associated with surgical technique, either from sewing the stomach over the band buckle or from microperforation of the stomach during surgery. Port and tubing problems include port migration, port infection, tubing disconnection, tubing kink, and port leak. These mechanical problems require surgical repair to maintain a functional device for weight loss.

Esophageal dilation may be an indication for band removal in patients who cannot tolerate restriction. DeMaria and associates [21] raised concerns about the possible long-term deleterious effects of long-term dilatation. In response to this, Fielding et al [31] have assessed follow-up results for complication, band removal, weight loss, and comorbidity reduction in patients with LAGB performed in 1998 by perigastric technique, and in 2000 by pars-flaccida technique, offering patients in 1998 a barium esophagram to assess dilatation. One hundred and twenty-three patients who had mean BMI 44.5 kg/m^2 had LAGB in 1998, and 162 who had mean BMI 44 had LAGB in 2000. Patient follow-up at mean 67 months was 88% for 1998 and 94% at 34 months for 2000. Mean excess weight loss (EWL) for 1998 was 51.2%, with mean BMI 31.9. Slip occurred in 9.5% of patients in 1998, compared with 4.3% in 2000 ($P < 0.01$). Only 1 of 34 patients had esophageal dilatation on barium esophagram. This dilatation completely resolved after band deflation.

Weight loss

There have now been more than 120,000 LAGBs placed, and there are numerous favorable early results published with 2- and 3-year follow-up. The one prospective randomized trial between LAGB and VBG [32], with 30 patients in each group, showed 6-month weight loss to be 50% EWL versus 87% EWL respectively, although 6-month data are meaningless. There are no long-term data from prospectively controlled studies. Early reports at 2 and 3 years suggested weight loss of 55% to 60% EWL (Table 1). Weight loss after LAGB is gradual and steady for up to 3 years, after which a steady plateau of 51% to 56% EWL is maintained out to 5 years. The purely restrictive nature of the operation results in daily caloric intake between 800 and 1200 for women and 1200 to 1500 for men, and thus a 1 to 2 lb per day weight loss is achieved. Average weight losses at years 1, 2, 3, 5 and 6 are 44.7%, 54.9%, 57.5%, 53%, and 57%, respectively (see Table 1).

Table 1
Outcomes of LAP-BAND System: % excess weight loss

Study	N	1 year	2 years	3 years	4 years	5 years	6 years	7 years
Dargent 1999 [30]	500	56	65	64				
Fielding 1999 [7]	335	52						
Allen 2001 [11]	60			65				
O'Brien 2002 [12]	709	47	52	53	52	54	57	
Vertruyen 2002 [29]	543	38	61	62	58	53		52
Rubenstein 2002 [34]	63	39	46.6	53.6				
Ren 2002 [35]	115	41.6						
Belachew 2002 [13]	763	40	50	50–60				

This has been further supported by more recent data at 5, 6, 7, and 8 years (Table 2). O'Brien and Dixon [16] have data on 1120 laparoscopic band patients at 6 years, with BMI falling from 46 to 30 kg/m^2, and 54% EWL. Weiner and coworkers [17] have 8-year data on 984 patients who had BMI 47, showing 57% EWL. Fielding and Duncombe [19] have 2110 bands, BMI 47, with 50% EWL at 6 years. A combined series from Europe [18] of 5827 patients who had a BMI of 46 has BMI 31 at 5 years. Steffen and coauthors [33] prospectively followed 824 patients after LAGB to 5 years (97% follow-up) and found that 83% achieved and maintained greater than 50% EWL. The second dominant theme of these longer-term follow-ups is that the laparoscopic band is effective.

Early experience in the United States was less satisfactory. In contrast to these positive international data, a small US series based around patients in the early FDA trial reported very high rates of band removal, correlating this with significant incidence of esophageal dilatation. DeMaria et al [30] reported high band-failure rates and band removal, in a series of perigastric bands that were infrequently adjusted. This obviously raised concerns about the long-term safety and efficacy of the LAGB in the US population, and had a profound effect on the perception of LAGB in the United States.

Results from more recent US experience more closely match those from abroad, however. Rubenstein [34] has reported on patients after having 54% EWL at 3 years follow-up. Subsequently, Ren et al [35] first showed that application of techniques used in Australia delivered comparable results. More recently, Ren, Weiner and Allen [36] reviewed their experience from May 2001 to December 2002 with 445 patients having a BMI 49.6 kg/m^2 (35–92). These patients had been treated as described above, with pars-flaccida technique, a loose band, and with slow steady adjustments performed in the office. There was one death (0.2%). At 1-year follow up, this cohort of patients had 44% EWL.

Patient attitudes

There can be little doubt that LAGB offers effective early weight loss, and that it is a safe procedure for morbidly obese individuals. This makes it very

Table 2
Mid-term follow-up LAGB (5–8 years)

Author	N	Followup years	Start BMI	Mortality	% EWL	BMI
O'Brien [16]	1120	6	46	0		31
Angrissani [9]	1265	5	44	0.5		
Fielding [19]	2110	6	47	0.05	50	31
Steffen [33]	825	5			57	
Europe	5827	5	46	0.2		31
Weiner [17]	984	8	47	0	57	
Vertruyen [29]	543	7			52	

attractive to many obese patients who would otherwise not come forward for surgery. Given the safety advantage and its effectiveness as a weight-loss tool, the LAGB is an attractive proposition for obese patients and their physicians. Two recent surveys have looked at why patients come forward for laparoscopic band surgery. The first [37], from Australia, showed that the dominant reason for surgery was ill health and fear of deteriorating future health, well in excess of concerns for appearance and fitness. Another combined study of 485 patients from New York and Australia [38] found that in both countries safety was the dominant reason people had come forward for LAGB.

Comorbidity resolution

The health benefits attendant on the weight loss that follows bariatric surgery are well known. They are the platform upon which the National Institutes of Health (NIH) guidelines for bariatric surgery have been created [39]. Reduction in multiple comorbidities has been well documented after LAGB surgery. O'Brien and coworkers [40] observed that after LAGB, patients experienced 74% improvement or resolution of dyslipidemia, 94% resolution of obstructive sleep apnea, 55% resolution of hypertension [41,42], 100% improvement of asthma, and 76% resolution with 14% improvement in gastroesophageal reflux [43–45]. In a study of 295 patients, Frigg et al [46] found that at 4 years, LAGB resulted in 54% EWL and 58% resolution of hypertension, 75% resolution of diabetes, and 79% resolution of reflux. There are no studies at this time that prospectively compare the outcomes of LAGB to nonsurgical medical management.

The role of LAGB surgery in the elimination of diabetes has recently been described. Dixon and O'Brien [47,48] reviewed 254 patients at surgery and 1 year. Thirty-nine patients were diabetics on medication. At 1 year, BMI fell from 46 to 36 kg/m^2, and weight fell from 128 kg to 101 kg, representing 44% EWL. The study showed a 50% increase in insulin sensitivity, from 16% to 25%, and a recovery of beta cell function. This was particularly beneficial in younger patients who had been diabetic for less than 5 years. Dolan and colleagues [48,49] reviewed 88 diabetic laparoscopic band patients, including 11 on insulin, with a 2-year follow-up. At 2 years, there was 51% EWL, and BMI fell from 47 to 34 kg/m^2. Seventy-four percent of patients on oral hypoglycaemic agents and 55% of patients on insulin were off all treatment by 6 months. The best predictor of cessation of therapy was 30% EWL.

Weight loss following LAGB surgery has a major impact on Type II diabetes mellitus, with resolution or improvement of diabetes in 80.8% of patients, as reflected by meta-analysis. In Buchwald and coauthors' meta-analysis [50], the control of diabetes with LAGB was 47.9% (95% confidence, 29.1–66.7), in contrast to that following RYGB, which was 83.7% (77.3–90.1); this was associated with a higher percentage EWL in the

RYGB group 68.2% (56.7–74.8) in contrast to the LAGB patients 47.5% (40.7–50.2). It has been suggested that the gastric bypass may provide control of diabetes through the early entry of food into the small intestine.

Follow-up

In their landmark 1995 paper, Pories and coworkers [51] showed that, with high levels of follow-up, good weight loss after RYGB is maintainable, and there is marked elimination of diabetes. Their degree of follow-up has not been widely replicated with gastric bypass, due perhaps to the transient nature of the modern population, with patients traveling great distances to the surgeon of their choice, and to the fact that there is little that can actually be modified by follow-up except discussion of eating habits and maintenance of nutrition. This group is much more difficult to follow, and follow-up rates of 60% to 80% are more typical. A recent report of 240 diabetics in a series of 1160 gastric bypasses from a dedicated bariatric service [52] described follow-up of 80% at mean follow-up of only 19.7 months (6–54 months).

Follow-up is a key ingredient for the success of LAGB surgery. There has been little in the literature actually defining outcome dependant on follow-up. Shen and coauthors [53] have recently produced data on differential rates of follow-up assessing outcome after LAGB. At their institution, in the first year of follow-up, band surgery patients were followed every 4 weeks and RYGB patients every 3 months. The number of follow-up visits for each patient was calculated, and 50% compliance on follow-up and weight loss was compared. Between October 2000 and December 2002, 216 LAGBs and 139 RYGBs were performed. Of these patients, 186 LAGBs were available for 1-year follow-up (86%). At 1 year, EWL for LAGB was 44.5%. Seventy percent returned six or fewer times, and achieved 42% EWL. Fifty-six patients returned more than 6 times and had 50% EWL ($P = 0.005$).

This early experience with LAGB in New York at 1 year confirms, for the first time, the importance of follow-up in maximizing outcome. Fielding and Duncombe [31] recently confirmed the importance of effective follow-up in a series of 197 bands performed in a closed community in Cairns, Australia. They had follow-up of 97% at a mean of 27 months, with a mean 57% EWL, maintained out to 6 years, with an average of five visits per year. There was almost complete resolution of comorbidity at 2 years in this community.

Band removal

All bariatric procedures carry the possibility of failure or patient intolerance. LAGBs are typically removed due to failed weight loss, band erosion, or uncontrolled symptoms of reflux esophagitis or dysphagia. This seems to occur at a rate of 3% to 6% in most large series. The LAGB has a real advantage in its ability to be easily removed by laparoscopy, and easy conversion to alternate procedures. Patients tend to be converted to either RYGB or BPD. Several authors have described RYGB to salvage failed LAGB [54–57]. None of these relatively small series describes any particular difficulty in performing the conversion. Dolan and Fielding [58] examined the failure rate with LAGB and results of band removal with BPDS ± DS for insufficient weight loss or a complication. The band was removed in 85 (5.9%) of 1439 patients, most commonly for persistent dysphagia and recurrent slippage. The removal rate and slippage rate decreased from 10.8% and 14.2% to 2.8% and 1.3%, respectively, following introduction of the pars-flaccida technique. Mean percentage EWLs 12 months following open BPD, laparoscopic BPD, open BPDDS and laparoscopic BPDDS were 44%, 37%, 35%, and 18%, respectively. The authors found that removal of the band with synchronous BPD or BPDDS can be performed laparoscopically. Favretti first described addition of the distal BPD-style bypass to a band for failed weight loss, leaving the band to control hunger. Himpens et al [59] described adding a band to a failed gastric bypass. Slater and Fielding [60] found identical results, showing that addition of a band to a failed BPD or a bypass to a failed band delivers excellent weight loss.

The advent of the 11-cm Vanguard (Inamed Health, Santa Barbara, California) band has expanded the possibilities in management of failed bands due to dysphagia. These bands are primarily indicated for hugely obese men, but have a place in this setting, and also in banding failed RYGB or BPD. Dargent [61] was the first to delineate the different possibilities. In a series of 1180 LAGBs performed since 1995, 67 (5.6%) were removed, and only 5 were converted to a different procedure. The remainder were repositioned, replaced for mechanical failure or erosion, or replaced with an 11-cm band.

Summary

Only a fraction of morbidly obese patients have come forward for bariatric surgery. This article confirms that LAGB is a safe, effective primary weight-loss operation for morbidly obese patients The LAGB offers a simple, genuinely minimally invasive approach, with the potential to be attractive to many more patients. The key questions are whether it is effective in the long term and whether it is safe. The midterm data confirm that the laparoscopic band is an effective tool. LAGB surgery is safe, and the change to the pars-flaccida approach will lead to even higher patient satisfaction and lower incidence of band removal. So far, LAGB is living up to its early promise as an effective, minimally invasive bariatric procedure.

References

[1] Belechew M, Legrand MJ, Defechereux TH, et al. Laparoscopic adjustable silicone gastric banding in the treatment of morbid obesity. A preliminary report. Surg Endosc 1994;8(11): 1354–6.

[2] De Luca M, de Wirra C, Formato. A laparotomic versus laparoscopic lap band: 4 year resultswith early and intermediate complications. Obes Surg 2000;10:266–8.

[3] De Wit L, Mathis-Vliegen L, Hey L, et al. Open vs laparoscopic adjustable gastric banding in a prospective trial for the treatment of morbid obesity. Ann Surg 1999;230:800–5.

[4] Suter M, Giusti V, Heraief E, et al. Early results of laparoscopic gastric bypass compared with open VBG. Obes Surg 1999;9:374–80.

[5] Chapman AE, Kiroff G, Game P, et al. Laparoscopic adjustable gastric banding in the treatment of obesity: a systematic literature review. Surgery 2004;135(3):326–51.

[6] O'Brien PE, Brown WA, Smith A, et al. Prospective study of a laparoscopically placed, adjustable gastric band in the treatment of morbid obesity. Br J Surg 1999;86(1): 113–8.

[7] Fielding GA, Rhodes M, Nathanson LK. Laparoscopic gastric banding for morbid obesity. Surgical outcome in 335 cases. Surg Endosc 1999;13(6):550–4.

[8] Spivak H, Anwar F, Burton S, et al. The LAP-BAND system in the United States: one surgeon's experience with 271 patients. Surg Endosc 2004;18(2):198–202.

[9] Angrisani L, Alkilani M, Basso N, et al. Laparoscopic Italian experience with the LAP-BAND. Obes Surg 200;11(3):307–10.

[10] Fox SR, Fox KM, Srikanth MS, et al. The LAP-BAND system in a North American population. Obes Surg 2003;13(2):275–80.

[11] Allen J, Coleman M, Fielding GA. Lessons learned from laparoscopic gastric banding for morbid obesity. Am J Surg 2001;182(1):10–4.

[12] O'Brien PE, Dixon JB, Brown W, et al. The laparoscopic adjustable gastric band (LAP-BAND): a prospective study of medium-term effects on weight, health and quality of life. Obes Surg 2002;12:652–60.

[13] Belachew M, Belva PH, Desaive C. Long-term results of laparoscopic adjustable gastric banding for the treatment of morbid obesity. Obes Surg 2002;12:564–8.

[14] Favretti F, Cadiere GB, Segato G, et al. Laparoscopic banding: selection and technique in 830 patients. Obes Surg 2002;12(3):385–90.

[15] Sarker S, Herold K, Creech S, et al. Early and late complications following laparoscopic adjustable gastric banding. Am Surg 2004;70:146–9.

[16] O'Brien PE, Dixon JB. LAP-BAND: outcomes and results. J Laparoendosc Adv Surg Tech A 2003;13(4):265–70.

[17] Weiner R, Blanco-Eugert R, Weiner R, et al. Outcome after laparoscopic adjustable gastric banding—8 years experience. Obes Surg 2003;13(3):427–34.

[18] O'Brien PE, Dixon JB. Weight loss and early and late complications—the international experience. Am J Surg 2002;184(6B):42S–5S.

[19] Fielding GA, Duncombe JE. Clinical and radiological follow up of a cohort of laparoscopic adjustable gastric bands from 1998. Obes Surg, in press.

[20] Angrisani L, Furbetta F, Doldi SB, et al. LAP-BAND adjustable gastric banding system: the Italian experience with 1863 patients operated on over 6 years. Surg Endosc 2003; 17(3):409–12.

[21] DeMaria EJ, Sugerman HJ, Meador JG, et al. High failure rate after laparoscopic adjustable silicone gastric banding for treatment of morbid obesity. Ann Surg 2001;233(6):809–18.

[22] Fernandez AZ Jr, DeMaria EJ, Tichansky DS, et al. Experience with over 3000 open and laparoscopic bariatric procedures: multivariate analysis of factors related to mortality and leak. Surg Endosc 2004;18(2):193–7.

[23] Flumm DR, Dellinger EP. Impact of gastric bypass operation on survival: a population-based analysis. J Am Coll Surg 2004;199:543–51.

[24] Laker S, Weiner M, Hajiseyedjavadi H, et al. Objective comparison of complications resulting from laparoscopic bariatric surgery. Surg Endosc 2004;18:5.

[25] Biertho L, Steffen R, Ricklin T, et al. Laparoscopic gastric bypass versus laparoscopic adjustable gastric banding: a comparative study of 1,200 cases. J Am Coll Surg 2003;197(4): 536–44.

[26] Fisher BL. Comparison of recovery time after open and laparoscopic gastric bypass and laparoscopic adjustable banding. Obes Surg 2004;14(1):67–72.

[27] Dolan K, Hatzifotis M, Newbury L, et al. A comparison of laparoscopic adjustable gastric banding and biliopancreatic diversion in superobesity. Obes Surg 2004;14:165–9.

[28] Ren CJ, Fielding GA. Laparoscopic adjustable gastric banding: surgical technique. J Laparoendosc Adv Surg Tech A 2003;13:257–63.

[29] Vertruyen M. Experience with LAP-BAND system up to 7 years. Obes Surg 2002;12:569–72.

[30] Dargent J. Laparoscopic adjustable gastric banding: lessons from the first 500 patients in a single institution. Obes Surg 1999;9:446–52.

[31] Fielding G, Duncombe J. Weight loss and clinical outcomes after laparoscopic adjustable gastric banding in a stable population in Northern Australia, with 97% follow-up. Med J Aust, in press.

[32] Ashy AR, Merdad AA. A prospective study comparing vertical banded gastroplasty versus laparoscopic adjustable gastric banding in the treatment of morbid and super-obesity. Int Surg 1998;83(2):108–10.

[33] Steffen R, Biertho L, Ricklin T, et al. Laparoscopic Swedish adjustable gastric banding: a five-year prospective study. Obes Surg 2003;13(3):404–11.

[34] Rubenstein RB. Laparoscopic adjustable gastric banding at a US center with up to 3-year follow-up. Obes Surg 2002;12(3):380–4.

[35] Ren CJ, Horgan S, Ponce J. US experience with the LAP-BAND system. Am J Surg 2002; 184(6B):46S–50S.

[36] Ren CJ, Weiner M, Allen JW. Favorable early results of gastric banding for morbid obesity: the American experience. Surg Endosc 2004;18(3):543–6.

[37] Libeton M, Dixon JB, Laurie C, et al. Patient motivation for bariatric surgery: characteristics and impact on outcomes. Obes Surg 2004;14(3):392–8.

[38] Ren CJ, Cabrera I, Rajaram K, et al. Factors influencing patient choice for bariatric surgery procedure. Obes Surg, in press.

[39] National Institutes of Health Consensus Development Conference Gastrointestinal surgery for severe obesity. Obes Surg 1991;1:257–66.

[40] O'Brien PE, Dixon JB, Smith A. The laparoscopic adjustable gastric band: a prospective study of medium term effects on weight, health and quality of life. Obes Surg 2002;12: 652–60.

[41] Dixon JB, Dixon ME, O'Brien PE. Depression in association with severe obesity: changes with weight loss. Arch Intern Med 2003;163(17):2058–65.

[42] Dixon JB, O'Brien PE. Changes in comorbidities and improvements in quality of life after LAP-BAND placement. Am J Surg 2002;184:51S–4S.

[43] Dixon JB, Chapman L, O'Brien P. Marked improvement in asthma after LAP-BAND surgery for morbid obesity. Obes Surg 1999;9(4):385–9.

[44] Dolan K, Finch R, Fielding G. Laparoscopic gastric banding and crural repair in the obese patient with a hiatal hernia. Obes Surg 2003;13(5):772–5.

[45] Dixon JB, O'Brien PE. Gastroesophageal reflux in obesity: the effect of LAP-BAND placement. Obes Surg 1999;9:527–31.

[46] Frigg A, Peterli R, Peters T, et al. Reduction in co-morbidities 4 years after laparoscopic adjustable gastric banding. Obes Surg 2004;14(2):216–23.

[47] Dixon JB, O'Brien P. Weight loss after gastric band improves insulin sensitivity and arrests beta cell loss. Diabet Med 2003;20:127–34.

[48] Dolan K, Bryant R, Fielding GA. Treating diabetes in the morbidly obese by laparoscopic gastric banding. Obes Surg 2003;13:439–43.

[49] Dixon JB, O'Brien PE. Health outcomes of severely obese type 2 diabetic subjects 1 year after laparoscopic adjustable silicone gastric banding. Diabetes Care 2002;25:358–63.

[50] Buchwald, et al. Bariatric surgery: a systemic review and meta-analysis. JAMA 2004;292: 1724–57.

[51] Pories WJ, Swanson MS, MacDonald KG, et al. Who would have thought it? An operation proves to be the most effective therapy for adult-onset diabetes mellitus. Ann Surg 199;222(3):339–50.

[52] Schauer PR, Burguera B, Ikramuddin S, et al. Effect of laparoscopic Roux-en Y gastric bypass on type 2 diabetes mellitus. Ann Surg 2003;238(4):467–84 [discussion: 484–5].

[53] Shen R, Dugay G, Cabrera I, et al. Impact of patient follow-up on weight loss after bariatric surgery. Obes Surg 2004;14(4):514–9.

[54] Suter M, Giusti V, Heraief E, et al. Band erosion after laparoscopic gastric banding: occurrence and results after conversion to Roux-en-Y gastric bypass. Obes Surg 2004;14: 381–6.

[55] Westling A, Ohrvall M, Gustavsson S. Roux-en-Y gastric bypass after previous unsuccessful gastric restrictive surgery. J Gastrointest Surg 2002;6:206–11.

[56] Weber M, Muller M, Michel JM, et al. Laparoscopic Roux-en-Y gastric bypass, but not rebanding, as rescue procedure for patients with failed laparoscopic gastric banding. Ann Surg 2003;238:827–33.

[57] Kothari SN, DeMaria EJ, Sugerman HJ, et al. Laparoscopic band failure: conversion to gastric bypass and their preliminary outcomes. Surgery 2002;131:625–9.

[58] Dolan K, Fielding GA. Biliopancreatic diversion following failure of laparoscopic adjustable gastric banding. Surg Endosc 2004;18(1):60–3.

[59] Hempens JM, Rogge F, Leman G, et al. Laproscopic adjustable band after Roux-en-Y bypass. Obes Surg 2001;11:528–31.

[60] Slater GH, Fielding GA. Combined laparoscopic adjustable gastric banding and BPD after failed bariatric surgery. Obes Surg 2004;14:677–82.

[61] Dargent J. Surgical treatment of morbid obesity by adjustable gastric band: the case for a conservative strategy in the case of failure—a 9 year series. Obes Surg 2004;14:986–90.

ELSEVIER
SAUNDERS

Surg Clin N Am 85 (2005) 141–149

SURGICAL
CLINICS OF
NORTH AMERICA

Laparoscopic biliopancreatic diversion with duodenal switch

Michel Gagner, MD, FRCS, FACS*,
Ronald Matteotti, MD

*Department of Surgery, New York Presbyterian Hospital,
Joan and Stanford I. Weill Medical College of Cornell University,
525 East 68th Street, New York, NY 10021, USA*

From the clinical experience gained in open biliopancreatic diversions, laparoscopy has been used recently in a large effort to improve some debilitating wound and respiratory complications. This article summarizes the current literature on this subject and present the authors' approach to the superobese and high-risk morbidly obese patient. Biliopancreatic diversion (BPD) described by Scopinaro et al in 1979 [1] remains one of the most effective procedures for treatment of morbidly obese patients, especially those who have a body mass index (BMI) of over 50 kg/m². Satisfactory weight loss is achieved, with an acceptably low rate of long-term nutritional complications. Further modifications by Hess and coauthors and Marceau and colleagues [2–4], mainly sleeve gastrectomy and duodenal switch (BPD/DS), have significantly diminish the more severe complications of BPD: dumping syndrome-related problems, ulcerogenicity, hypoproteinemia, and hypocalcemia. The antrum, pylorus, first part of the duodenum, lesser curvature of the stomach, and vagal nerve integrity are spared, allowing normal eating behavior. The restrictive part of the procedure consists of creating a sleeve-shaped gastric pouch of 100 to 150 mL volume. The sleeve gastrectomy is created with the sequential firing of linear cutting staplers, starting at 8 to 10 cm proximal to the pylorus and proceeding toward the angle of His. The next steps involve the creation of a 150-cm alimentary limb and a common channel of 100 cm.

* Corresponding author.
E-mail address: mig2016@med.cornell.edu (M. Gagner).

0039-6109/05/$ - see front matter © 2005 Elsevier Inc. All rights reserved.
doi:10.1016/j.suc.2004.10.003   surgical.theclinics.com

Appraisal of literature

There has been no randomized controlled trial comparing either BPD or BPD/DS and other bariatric operations. Four cohort studies, 2 case-control studies, and 10 case studies showed excellent weight loss after BPD (level of evidence, 2A, grade B). One case-control study and three case studies showed weight loss after BPD/DS (level of evidence, 3B, grade B). Therefore, randomized controlled trials comparing malabsorptive procedures (BPD, BPD/DS) with other bariatric procedures are needed. Only 2 case studies have been reported for BPD/DS and 3 case studies in laparoscopic BPD. In 1999, Gagner and colleagues [5,6] established for the first time the feasibility of a laparoscopic approach to perform a BPD/DS in a porcine model, and after these positive results, Gagner [6] started to use this procedure in patients in early July 1999. Only a few surgical groups performed this operation laparoscopically [7–13]. These procedures are complex and technically more difficult to perform, especially the upper anastomosis, and they involve closure of a duodenal stump notorious for complications. All studies are retrospective and no prospective randomized studies are available comparing laparoscopic gastric bypass and BPD or BPD/DS. The literature available now reports on a total of 467 patients, and a majority of procedures were performed using a hand-assisted technique [13].

The first case of laparoscopic BPD (with DS modification) was performed in July 1999 by Gagner, and the series of 40 consecutive patients who had a median BMI of 60 kg/m^2 (range 42–85 kg/m^2) showed that 1 patient underwent conversion to laparotomy (2.5%), that median length of stay was 4 days (range 3–210 days), and that there was one 30-day mortality (2.5%) [7,14]. Major morbidities occurred in 6 patients (15%), and an estimated excess weight loss of 58% at 9 months occurred. Baltasar and coauthors [8] of Alicante, Spain, with successful performance of 16 cases, published the second case study with a postoperative stay varying between 5 and 8 days. Since then, several technical modifications have been presented at the last congress of the American Society for Bariatric Surgery. Smith and associates [15] demonstrated that hand-sewn duodeno-ileostomy can be performed in the same time as a stapled technique with low complications. Sudan and Sudan [16] used an intracorporeal robotic assisted technique for laparoscopic DS, which was found to be very time-consuming. A hand-assisted technique was developed to facilitate the learning curve of laparoscopic DS with the addition of laparoscopic cholecystectomy and appendectomy, by Rabkin et al [13] in San Francisco.

For laparoscopic BPD, a series of 40 patients [9] was performed in Belo Horizonte, Brazil between July 2000 and April 2001. Patients had an average BMI of 43.6 kg/m^2, there were no conversions, and cholecystectomy was added. Mortality was seen in 2.5% of patients, and major morbidity was seen in 12.5% of patients (pulmonary emboli, gastrointestinal bleeding, and fistula [9,11]). The mean excess weight loss at 10 months was 90%. Scopinaro and coworkers [12] have also developed a laparoscopic modification to his operation in 26 patients who had a mean BMI of 43 kg/m^2. The weight loss was reported to be the same as with his open procedure. The anastomosis was fashioned using an endoGIA, side to side, for a larger gastrojejunostomy needed for standard BPD [12]. Domene and associates [10] from Sao Paulo, Brazil reported successfully on gastric preserving laparoscopic BPD in 12 female patients, which is really a modified very distal gastric bypass.

A recent analysis of the 467 patients operated on and patient demographics is presented in Table 1. The mean age in these studies is 39, with a preponderance of female patients (63.5%) and preoperative mean BMI was 47.3 kg/m^2. Two out of these five studies reported high percentages of associated comorbidities, with hypertension, diabetes mellitus, degenerative joint disease, or sleep apnea [7,9]. Specific information about technical details and conversions are presented in Table 2. Fewer data are available concerning the conservative BPD performed laparoscopically; indeed, two groups [9,12] performed a BPD using a classical distal gastrectomy instead of preserving the pylorus, which is a main goal of duodenal switch [7–9,13]. The conversion rate varies widely, and is highest in the series of Scopinaro et al [12] at 26%; a mean of 6.1% is reported for the entire 467 patients. Scopinaro's group became familiar with the laparoscopic principles only recently, and this may explain a much higher conversion rate. If we look at the proximal anastomosis, a widespread of technical possibilities are used. Whereas Gagner and his group [6,7] proposed to use a 21- or 25-mm circular stapler (CEEA, US Surgical Corporation, Norwalk, Connecticut) to perform the proximal anastomosis, other groups are performing the gastro- or duodeno-ileostomy using linear staplers or even a handsewn technique (Fig. 1). Scopinaro's group [12] inappropriately used the circular stapler technique for the performance of a gastro-ileostomy, when it was only described for a duodeno-ileostomy. This led to an unacceptably high rate of stenosis. Technical problems were

Table 1
Laparoscopic BPD and DS: patient demographics

Study	Year of publication	Study type	N	Mean age	Female (%)	Mean BMI	Comorbidities (%)
Gagner et al [6,7]	2000	retrospective	40	43	70	60	75
Paiva et al [9,11]	2002	retrospective	40	39	72	43.6	95
Scopinaro et al [12]	2002	retrospective	26	36	73	43	NR
Baltasar et al [8]	2002	retrospective	16	36.5	16	>40	NR
Rabkin et al [13][a]	2003	retrospective	345	43	87	50	NR
Total/mean	-	-	467	39	63.5	47.3	-

Abbreviation: NR, not recorded.
[a] Hand-assisted series.

Table 2
Laparoscopic BPD and DS: intraoperative data

Study	Op type: BPD or DS	Conversion (%)	Op. time (min)	Upper anastomosis technique	Pouch (ml)	Reop (%)	App.	Chol.	Liver biopsy
Gagner et al [6,7]	DS	2.5	210	circular	175	7.5	NR	no	NR
Paiva et al [9,11]	BPD	0	210	Linear	350	0	NR	yes	NR
Scopinaro et al [12]	BPD	26	240	Linear	300	NR	NR	NR	NR
Baltasar et al [8]	DS	NR	232	handsewn	NR	12.5	NR	NR	NR
Rabkin et al [13][a]	DS	2	201	circular	124	4	yes	yes	yes
Total/mean	-	6.1	218.6	-	190	4.8	-	-	-

Abbreviations: App, appendectomy; Chol, cholecystectomy; NR, not recorded; OP, operative; Reop, reoperation.
[a] Hand-assisted series.

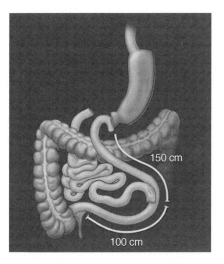

Fig. 1. Laparoscopic BPD/DS with a common channel of 100 cm and an alimentary limb of 150 cm. A duodeno-ileostomy end-to-side antecolic with mesenteric defects closed has been performed with a circular stapler EEA #21.

addressed, of course, by the appropriate technique for this anastomosis: a linear stapled, long and widely patent, side-to-side gastro-ileostomy. Another point that is not well defined in the literature is the performance of an additional cholecystectomy to prevent gallstones, or removal of the appendix or liver biopsy to assess the initial damage of this organ. Only Paiva and coauthors [9] and Rabkin and associates [13] are performing routine cholecystectomy routinely; only Rabkin and his group remove the appendix and take a liver biopsy. Looking at the postoperative course of these patients (Table 3), we see a mean excessive weight loss of 72% during a mean follow-up of approximately 12 months. Rabkin et al [13] report in their series a follow-up of 24 months, with a mean excessive weight loss of 91%. A reoperation rate of 4.8% is very acceptable, and an early

Table 3
Laparoscopic BPD and DS: follow-up data

Study	Follow-up (months)	Reoperation (%)	LOS # (days)	Complication early (%)	Deaths (%)	EWL (%)
Gagner et al [6,7]	9	7.5	4	15	5	58
Paiva et al [9,11]	NR	0	4.3	12.5	2.5	NR
Scopinaro et al [12]	12	NR	NR	NR	0	68
Baltasar et al [8]	NR	12.5	5.8	NR	0	NR
Rabkin et al [13][a]	24	4.1	3	2.6	0	91
Total/mean	12	4.8	3.3	6	0.6	72

Abbreviations: EWL, excess weight loss; LOS, length of stay; NR, not recorded.
[a] Hand-assisted series.

complication rate of 6% was encountered for these high-risk patients. A length of hospital stay of 3.3 days using a laparoscopic approach is much lower when one compares it with a minimum of 5 days in a larger series of 701 patients using the open procedure [17]. The overall mortality of 0.6% was only reported by two groups [7,9], and was 5% and 2.5% respectively.

Two-stage procedure

In a more recent series, Kim et al [18] reported that laparoscopic DS achieved a greater degree of permanent weight loss in morbidly obese patients, with a lower morbidity rate of 13% and a mortality of 1.4%. When data were stratified based on body mass index (BMI), however, super-super morbidly obese patients (BMI $\geq$60 kg/m^2) had a 23% morbidity rate and a 6.5% mortality rate. Super-super morbidly obese patients are on the extreme end of the spectrum of morbid obesity, with all its ramifications. Though BPD/DS could achieve excellent weight loss with acceptable risks in obese patients, review of our open BPD/DS patients who had a BMI >60 kg/m^2 (n = 28) showed 17% morbidity and 3.5% mortality. A laparoscopic approach in this population is potentially beneficial from the cardiovascular, pulmonary, infectious and wound-healing points of view. Neither open nor laparoscopic one-stage approaches have been satisfactory in this group of patients. The authors have hypothesized that separating the restrictive and malabsorptive aspects of the procedure into two operative stages—laparoscopic sleeve gastrectomy and laparoscopic duodenoileostomy-ileoileostomy—would reduce the complication and mortality rates [19,20]. Between September 2000 and September 2001, 18 patients who had a BMI $\geq$60 kg/m^2 completed the two-stage laparoscopic BPD/DS. Thirteen women and five men with a median age of 41 years (25–56 years) were operated on. At the time of laparoscopic sleeve gastrectomy, the mean weight was 187 $\pm$ 26 kg, and the mean BMI was 65.8 $\pm$ 4.7 kg/m^2. Surgery resulted in a mean excess body weight loss (EBWL) of 30.5% $\pm$ 8.0 at 6 months. The median time interval between the operations was 196 days (71 to 321 days). The mean BMI at time of the second procedure was 50.7 $\pm$ 5.9 kg/m^2. The EBWL percentages at 3 weeks, 3 months, and 6 months were 42.0 $\pm$ 10.3%, 52.6 $\pm$ 9.0%, and 71.4 $\pm$ 7.5%, respectively. The median operative times for the first and second stages were 97 $\pm$ 28 and 141 $\pm$ 37.7 minutes. Hospital stay was a mean of 3 days each. Overall, there was no mortality, one wound infection (2.8%) and one Deep Vein Thrombosis (DVT) with transient hypoproteinemia (2.8%). Laparoscopic sleeve gastrectomy and interval laparoscopic duodenoileostomy-ileoileostomy are safe and effective procedures. There is a drastic reduction in the morbidity and mortality using this approach compared with our historical cohort. A two-stage laparoscopoic BPD/DS is an alternative to the traditional one-stage approach for super-super morbidly obese patients [19,20].

Laparoscopic reoperations

Revisional surgery for patients who have inadequate weight loss after diversion with DS is controversial. It has not yet been determined whether a common channel should be shortened or gastric pouch volume reduced. Because the revision of the distal anastomosis remains technically difficult and is associated with possible complications, our group turned its attention to the reduction of gastric sleeve volume [21]. This operation is more feasible and potential complications are less probable. We have recently preformed a "resleeve" on the stomach, in a 47-year-old woman who had previous laparoscopic DS with a 100 mL gastric pouch, 150 cm of alimentary limb, and 100 cm of common channel [22]. Before the operation, her weight was 170 kg and her BMI was 64 kg/m^2. She lost most of her excess weight within 17 months after surgery, and was regaining weight at 77 kg with a BMI at 29 kg/m2. An upper gastrointestinal series showed a markedly dilated upper gastric fundic pouch. Her second surgery consisted of a laparoscopic sleeve partial gastrectomy along the greater curvature, using endoGIA staplers with Bovine pericardium for reinforcement of the stapler line. No postoperative complications occurred and the patient was discharged the following day. Significant further weight reduction was noted within 5 months after surgery, with a weight of 63 kg and BMI of 24 kg/m^2. A repeat laparoscopic gastric sleeve resection is feasible and safe in inadequate weight loss after BPD/DS and results in further weight reduction.

New concepts

Finally, new concepts that several experienced surgeons have found shocking were introduced. Vassallo and colleagues [23] have proposed a somewhat modified concept, in which an open transitory gastroplasty with an absorbable band to provide a temporary restriction was added to an open duodenal switch, preserving entirely the stomach. Their study was published in 1997, and the operation was performed in 53 cases without diarrhea or protein deficiency. More recently, Mittenpergher and coauthors [24] from the University of Brescia in Italy have performed this open operation in 74 patients using a band of polydioxanone (PDS) to preserve the first 5 cm of duodenum, with an initial excess weight loss of 69.8% after 1 year, and 75.2% after 5 years. There was no mortality and there were no cases of hypoalbuminemia or diarrhea. Only 1 patient (1.3%) developed an anastomotic ulcer. After 5 years, these authors observed 2 cases (12.5%) of chronic hypochromic anemia and 1 case (6.2%) of hypocalcemia. A recent case in which the Vertical Banded Gastroplasty (VBG) was left intact and an open duodenal switch was added is somewhat similar in concept to the one we are proposing. This has not led to protein deficiencies with an additional EBWL of 36.4% [25]. Because some morbidity in the BPD is due to gastric resection, it has been replaced by an adjustable gastric banding, an easier procedure, to further reduce the complication rate. Cadiere and Favretti have been early proponents of adding laparoscopic duodenal switch to failed previous laparoscopic gastric banding. Gagner [26] preferred to do a laparoscopic duodenal switch with a sleeve gastrectomy at the time of laparoscopic gastric banding removal for those failures. In August 2001, Gagner and Steffen [27] from Berne, Switzerland performed laparoscopic adjustable gastric banding with duodenal switch (a 250-cm alimentary channel, and a 100-cm common channel) during the same operative time. All 5 patients were women, with a mean preoperative BMI of 52.2 kg/m^2 (40.6–64.4 kg/m^2). The operations were performed under laparoscopy in a mean 206 $\pm$ 35 minutes. There were no postoperative complications, infections, or conversions. Mean hospital stay was 8.8 days (8–11 days). After 5 months, BMI was 43.4 kg/m^2, with an EBWL of 30%. These data suggest that laparoscopic adjustable gastric banding with laparoscopic duodenal switch is feasible, with a low morbidity rate. This technique could combine the long-term weight loss of malabsorptive procedures with a low-morbidity, adjustable, restrictive procedure. This technique could be used in selected patients, but requires a larger study with longer follow-up.

Summary

Preliminary results demonstrate the feasibility and safety of laparoscopic biliopancreatic diversion with duodenal switch, knowing that the superobese patient carries a higher risk than the normal population or the regular obese patient [28]. Future studies with larger number of patients should be able to demonstrate the effectiveness of this procedure in reducing weight and comorbidities such as hyperlipidemia, hypertension, sleep apnea, and diabetes mellitus, an effectiveness that has been proven in the open approach.

There is currently poor evidence regarding this effectiveness, due to small case series and early follow-up [29]. Further research is needed to examine long-term efficacy, with a high priority given to randomized controlled trials.

References

[1] Scopinaro N, Gianetta E, Civalleri D, et al. Bilio-pancreatic bypass for obesity: II. Initial experience in man. Br J Surg 1979;66(9):618–20.
[2] Marceau P, Biron S, Bourque RA, et al. Biliopancreatic diversion with a new type of gastrectomy. Obes Surg 1993;3(1):29–35.
[3] Hess DS, Hess DW. Biliopancreatic diversion with a duodenal switch. Obes Surg 1998;8: 267–82.
[4] Marceau P, Hould FS, Simard S, et al. Biliopancreatic diversion with duodenal switch. World J Surg 1998;22(9):947–54.
[5] De Csepel J, Burpee S, Jossart G, et al. Laparoscopic biliopancreatic diversion with a duodenal switch for morbid obesity: a feasibility study in pigs. J Laparoendosc Adv Surg Tech A 2001;11(2):79–83.
[6] Gagner M, Patterson E. Laparoscopic biliopancreatic diversion with duodenal switch. Dig Surg 2000;17:547–66.

[7] Ren CJ, Patterson E, Gagner M. Early results of laparoscopic biliopancreatic diversion with duodenal switch: a case series of 40 consecutive patients. Obes Surg 2000;10(6):514–23 [discussion: 524].

[8] Baltasar A, Bou R, Miro J, et al. Laparoscopic biliopancreatic diversion with duodenal switch: technique and initial experience. Obes Surg 2002;12(2):245–8.

[9] Paiva D, Bernardes L, Suretti L. Laparoscopic biliopancreatic diversion for the treatment of morbid obesity: initial experience. Obes Surg 2001;11(5):619–22.

[10] Domene CE, Resera I, Ciongoli J. Derivacao biliopancreatica com preservacao gastrica videolaparoscopica-sistematizacao tecnica. Rev Col Bras Cir 2001;28(6):453–5.

[11] Paiva D, Bernardes L, Suretti L. Laparoscopic biliopancreatic diversion: technique and initial results. Obes Surg 2002;12:358–61.

[12] Scopinaro N, Marinari GM, Camerini G. Laparoscopic standard biliopancreatic diversion: technique and preliminary results. Obes Surg 2002;12(3):362–5.

[13] Rabkin RA, Rabkin JM, Metcalf B, et al. Laparoscopic technique for performing duodenal switch with gastric reduction. Obes Surg 2003;13(2):263–8.

[14] Feng JJ, Gagner M. Laparoscopic biliopancreatic diversion with duodenal switch. Semin Laparosc Surg 2002;9(2):125–9.

[15] Smith DC, Hendricks K, O'Reilly MJ. Laparoscopic biliopancreatic diversion with duodenal switch, with hand-sewn duodeno-ileostomy [abstract]. Obes Surg 2002;12:206.

[16] Sudan R, Sudan D. Development of a totally intracorporeal robotic assisted biliary pancreatic diversion with duodenal switch [abstract]. Obes Surg 2002;12:205.

[17] Anthone GJ, Lord RV, DeMeester TR, et al. The duodenal switch operation for the treatment of morbid obesity. Ann Surg 2003;238(4):618–27 [discussion: 627–8].

[18] Kim WW, Gagner M, Kini S, et al. Laparoscopic vs. open biliopancreatic diversion with duodenal switch: a comparative study. J Gastrointest Surg 2003;7(4):552–7.

[19] Gagner M, Chu CA, Inabnet WB, et al. Two-stage laparoscopic biliopancreatic diversion with duodenal switch: an alternative approach to super-super morbid obesity. Surg Endosc, in press.

[20] Regan JP, Inabnet WB, Gagner M, et al. Early experience with a two-stage laparoscopic Roux-en-Y gastric bypass as an alternative in the super-super obese patient. Obes Surg 2003; 13(6):861–4.

[21] Papachristou D, Fotiadis C, Baramily B, et al. Prevention of obesity in swine by longitudinal gastrectomy. Ann Chir 1988;42(5):357–9.

[22] Gagner M, Rogula T. Laparoscopic reoperative sleeve gastrectomy for poor weight loss after biliopancreatic diversion with duodenal switch. Obes Surg 2003;13(4):649–54.

[23] Vassallo C, Negri L, Della Valle A, et al. Biliopancreatic diversion with transitory gastroplasty preserving duodenal bulb: 3 years experience. Obes Surg 1997;7(1):30–3.

[24] Mittempergher F, Bruni T, Bruni O, et al. Billiopancreatic diversion with preservation of the duodenal bulb and transitory gastroplasty in the treatment of morbid obesity. Our experience. Ann Ital Chir 2002;73(2):137–42.

[25] Yashkov YI, Oppel TA, Shishlo LA, et al. Improvement of weight loss and metabolic effects of vertical banded gastroplasty by an added duodenal switch procedure. Obes Surg 2001; 11(5):635–9.

[26] De Csepel J, Quinn T, Pomp A, et al. Conversion to a laparoscopic biliopancreatic diversion with a duodenal switch for a failed laparoscopic adjustable silicone gastric banding. J Laparoendosc Adv Surg Tech A 2002;12(4):237–40.

[27] Gagner M, Steffen R, Biertho L, et al. Laparoscopic adjustable gastric banding with duodenal switch for morbid obesity. Technique and preliminary results. Obes Surg 2003; 13(3):444–9.

[28] Sekhar N, Gagner M. Complications of laparoscopic biliopancreatic diversion with duodenal switch. Curr Surg 2003;60(3):279–80.

[29] Gentileschi P, Kini S, Catarci M, et al. Evidence-based medicine: open and laparoscopic bariatric surgery. Surg Endosc 2002;16:736–44.

ELSEVIER
SAUNDERS

SURGICAL
CLINICS OF
NORTH AMERICA

Surg Clin N Am 85 (2005) 151–164

Minimally invasive surgery for gastric tumors

Seigo Kitano, MD, FACS*, Norio Shiraishi, MD

*Department of Surgery I, Faculty of Medicine, Oita University, 1-1 Idaigaoka,
Hasama-machi, Oita 879-55, Japan*

Gastric tumor, especially gastric cancer, remains one of the most common causes of cancer death in the world. The incidence of early gastric cancer has increased, however, with rapid advances in diagnostic instrumentation and the popularity of mass screening and individual examination. Because patients who have early gastric cancer have a low recurrence rate and a long survival period, attention should be directed to the quality of life (QOL) after surgery.

Laparoscopic cholecystectomy has clear advantages over open surgery, including early recovery of bowel function, early hospital discharge, and decreased pain [1,2]. Therefore, laparoscopic procedures have been adopted for the treatment of gastric tumor. Since Kitano et al's first report of successful laparoscopy-assisted distal gastrectomy (LADG) for early gastric cancer in 1994 [3], the number of laparoscopic surgeries for gastric cancer has increased, and several new laparoscopic procedures for specific gastric tumors, such as gastrointestinal submucosal tumor (GIST) and malignant lymphoma, have been developed [4,5]. Several studies of the short-term outcome of these procedures have been published, but there have been few evaluations of the long-term outcome.

In this article, the authors review the literature on the present status and outcomes of laparoscopic surgery for gastric tumor, mainly gastric cancer.

Development of laparoscopic gastric surgery

Laparoscopic surgery for gastric tumor is more common in Asian countries, especially Japan, than in Western countries because of the higher

---

* Corresponding author.
  E-mail address: kitano@med.oita-u.ac.jp (S. Kitano).

0039-6109/05/$ - see front matter © 2005 Elsevier Inc. All rights reserved.
doi:10.1016/j.suc.2004.09.004   surgical.theclinics.com

incidence of this tumor in Asian countries; however, laparoscopic surgery for gastric tumor has not yet achieved worldwide acceptance equal to that of laparoscopic colectomy for colon cancer.

Among gastric tumors, early-stage cancers have been considered the best candidates for laparoscopic surgery, and many new laparoscopic procedures for early gastric cancer have been developed since Kitano et al [3] first reported LADG in 1994 (Table 1). These laparoscopic procedures are categorized according to the extent of lymph node dissection: laparoscopic local resection without lymph node dissection, laparoscopic gastrectomy with lymph node dissection (D1, D1 + α, and D1 + β), and laparoscopic gastrectomy with extensive lymph node dissection (D2). By the latter half of the 1990s, laparoscopic procedures were also being used to treat advanced gastric cancer.

A national survey conducted by the Japan Society of Endoscopic Surgery (JSES) showed increasing use of laparoscopic procedures to treat gastric cancer in Japan (Fig. 1) [15]. During the period 1991 to 2001, 4552 patients underwent laparoscopic surgery for gastric cancer. The use of LADG with D1 + α or β lymph node dissection has increased rapidly, and this procedure now accounts for about 75% of all laparoscopic surgeries for gastric cancer.

Since the latter half of the 1990s, there have been multiple studies of the short-term outcomes of laparoscopic surgery, but there have been few randomized controlled trials or studies of long-term outcomes.

Laparoscopic local resection for gastric cancer

There are two procedures for laparoscopic local resection of early gastric cancer: laparoscopic wedge resection (LWR) by a lesion-lifting method, and intragastric mucosal resection (IGMR) [4,16].

Indications

Laparoscopic local resection is used to treat early gastric cancer without lymph node metastasis that is not a candidate for endoscopic mucosal resection (EMR) because of tumor size or location. Lymph node metastasis occurs in 2% to 5% of mucosal cancers and in 15% to 20% of submucosal cancers. Despite many reports, the pathological characteristics of early gastric cancer without lymph node metastasis remain controversial. Hyung and colleagues [17] observed that when lymphatic or blood vessel invasion was absent, there was no lymph node metastasis if the tumor was smaller than 2.5 cm and histologically differentiated, or smaller than 1.5 cm and histologically undifferentiated, regardless of the depth of gastric wall invasion. The Japanese Gastric Cancer Association guidelines define early gastric cancer without lymph node metastasis as mucosal cancer less than 2.0 cm in diameter, histologically differentiated, and without ulceration [18].

Table 1
Development of laparoscopic gastrectomy

Year	First author	Operation	Report
1994	Kitano S [3]	Laparoscopy-assisted Billroth-I gastrectomy (LADG)	Surg Endosc Laparosc Percutan Tech
1995	Watson DI [6]	Laparoscopic Billroth-II gastrectomy	Br J Surg
	Uyama I [7]	Laparoscopy-assisted proximal gastrectomy	Surg Laparosc Endosc
1997	Taniguchi S [8]	Laparoscopic pyrorus-preserving gastrectomy	Surg Laparosc Endosc
1999	Uyama I [9]	Laparoscopic total gastrectomy (D2) (for advanced cancer)	Gastric Cancer
	Ohki J [10]	Hand-assisted laparoscopic distal gastrectomy	Surg Endosc
	Kitano S [11]	Laparoscopy-assisted proximal gastrectomy, reconstruction by gastric tube	Surg Today
2001	Goh PM [12]	Laparoscopic radical gastrectomy (D2) (for advanced cancer)	Surg Endosc Laparosc Percutan Tech
	Uyama I [13]	Laparoscopic side-to-side esophagogastrostomy after proximal gastrectomy	Gastric Cancer
2002	Mochiki E [14]	Laparoscopically assisted total gastrectomy with jejunal interposition	Surg Endosc

Therefore, Ogami and coauthors, who developed LWR, proposed the following indications for LWR: preoperatively diagnosed mucosal cancer, elevated lesions less than 25 mm in diameter, or depressed lesions less than 15 mm in diameter without ulcer formation [4]. The pathological indications for IGMR are the same as those of LWR. The method chosen depends on

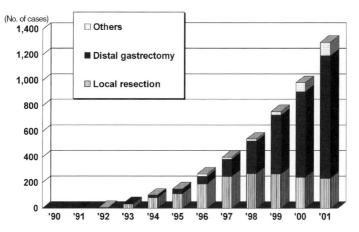

Fig. 1. Laparoscopic surgery was implemented for gastric cancer in 1991. The number of procedures totaled 4500 through 2001. (*From* Japan Society for Endoscopic Surgery. Nationwide survey on endoscopic surgery in Japan. Journal of Japan Society for Endoscopic Surgery 2002;7:500 [in Japanese]; with permission).

the location of the tumor. LWR is applied for cancer located on the anterior wall, lesser curvature, or greater curvature of the stomach; IGMR is applied for cancers on the posterior wall of the stomach or near the cardia or pylorus.

Techniques of laparoscopic wedge resection and intragastric mucosal resection

In both LWR and IGMR, intraoperative endoscopic observation is required to localize the cancer.

Laparoscopic wedge resection
LWR is performed as follows [4]:

(1) The gastric wall around the cancer is identified under both endoscopic and laparoscopic observation.
(2) The abdominal wall and gastric wall in the vicinity of lesion are pierced using a 12-G sheathed needle, and a small metal rod with a fine wire is introduced into the stomach through the outer sheath.
(3) After retracting the metal rod to lift the cancerous lesion, wedge resection at a sufficient distance from the metal rod is performed using a laparoscopic stapler.

Intragastric mucosal resection
IGMR consisted of the following procedures [16]:

(1) Three balloon trocars are placed in the gastric lumen, penetrating the abdomen and stomach wall.
(2) The stomach is insufflated with CO_2, and surgical instruments are introduced.
(3) Mucosal resection is performed with the use of forceps, electrocautery, and laser under both laparoscopic and endoscopic observation.
(4) After the resected specimen is extracted endoscopically, each trocar site in the stomach is closed under laparoscopic surgery.

Present status

Although LWR is popular in Japan for early gastric cancer, it is more commonly performed worldwide for the treatment of GIST. IGMR is not as popular in Japan or elsewhere because of the technical difficulty of the procedure.

According to the JSES [15], LWR was performed in Japan in 1428 cases and IGMR in 260 cases during the period 1991 to 2001. Endoscopic submucosal dissection (ESD), a recently developed EMR method [19], enables endoscopic en-bloc dissection of larger lesions. The use of LWR may decrease as the use of ESD increases. Kitagawas report [20] of the usefulness of sentinel node navigation before LWR will likely increase the use of LWR with sentinel node navigation.

Evaluation of laparoscopic wedge resection and intragastric mucosal resection

There are few reports on the short- and long-term outcomes of laparoscopic local resection. The reported outcomes are summarized in Table 2. In Ohgami's series of 111 cases [4] (LWR, n = 93; IGMR, n = 18), there were no major complications or mortality, and patients were discharged uneventfully in 4 to 8 days. There were no conversions to open surgery. The resected specimens had sufficient surgical margins horizontally (LWR, 15 ± 5 mm; IGMR, 8 ± 4 mm) and vertically. There were two recurrences (1.8%), both of which were found near the staple line 2 years after surgery and successfully treated by open gastrectomy and laser irradiation. Shimizu et al [21] reported the short-term outcome of 24 laparoscopic local resections (LWR, n = 20; IGMR, n = 4). One LWR and one IGMR were converted to open surgery. Operation time was 144 ± 34 and 298 ± 106 minutes for LWR and IGMR, respectively, and blood loss was 56 ± 94 and 33 ± 58 g, respectively. One patient suffered a complication (bleeding) after IGMR, and there were no complications after LWR. Hospital stay was 12 ± 4 and 16 ± 3 days after LWR and IGMR, respectively. In Kobayashi and coworkers [23] department, 18 laparoscopic local resections (LWR, n = 11; IGMR, n = 7) were performed. Four patients in the IGMR group were converted to open surgery. Histologic examination showed submucosal invasion in five patients, one of whom consequently underwent open gastrectomy.

Further evaluation of the outcomes of laparoscopic local resection is necessary; however, laparoscopic local resection seems to be safe and

Table 2
Evaluation of laparoscopic local resection for cancer

First author	Report	Cases (LWR/IGMR)	Advantage of LWR
Ohgami M.	Nippon Geka Gakkai Zasshi (2000) [4]	93/18 (case)	No major complication Sufficient surgical margin Recurrence in two cases
Shimizu S.	J Am Coll Surg (2003) [21]	20/4 (case)	Detailed histological examination Faster postoperative recover Fewer complications
Kobayashi T.	Surg Endosc Laparosc Percutan Tech (2003) [22]	11/7 (case)	Curative operation Safe procedures

curative when the appropriate indications are used. Precise preoperative and postoperative diagnosis is important.

Laparoscopic gastrectomy for gastric cancer

LADG is the most popular method of laparoscopic gastrectomy. The indications for proximal and total gastrectomy have recently been challenged.

Indications for laparoscopy-assisted distal gastrectomy

LADG for gastric cancer can be performed with perigastric lymph node dissection (D1 + α), additional lymph node dissection along the common hepatic artery (D1 + β), and extended lymph node dissection (D2). The extent of lymph node dissection necessary for the treatment of submucosal cancer is still controversial. Omote et al reported no lymph node metastasis from tumors of less than 300 um submucosal invasion and less than 3 cm in diameter [23]. Oizumi and coauthors [24] and Fujii and associates [25] found no metastasis in patients who have submucosal tumor less than 1 cm in diameter. Hyung and coauthors [17] proposed that D2 lymph node dissection is indicated for differentiated submucosal cancers of more than 2.5 cm in diameter and for undifferentiated submucosal cancers of more than 1.5 cm. Yasuda et al [5] showed that submucosal cancers measuring 1 to 4 cm in diameter were sometimes positive for lymph node metastasis but rarely for extragastric lymph node metastasis, and concluded that D1 + α is the optimal lymph node dissection level for these submucosal cancers. The Japanese Gastric Cancer Association guidelines determine the optimal lymph node dissection level for early gastric cancer on the basis of preoperative diagnosis, as follows: D1 + α for mucosal cancer for which EMR is not indicated and for histologically differentiated submucosal cancer less than 1.5 cm in diameter; D1 + β for submucosal cancer without preoperatively diagnosed lymph node metastasis (N0) for which D1 + α is not indicated, and for early cancer less than 2.0 cm in diameter with preoperatively diagnosed perigastric lymph node metastasis (N1); D2 for early N1 cancer more 2.0 cm in diameter, early cancer with extended lymph node metastasis (N2 +), and advanced cancer.

Techniques of laparoscopy-assisted distal gastrectomy

To identify the oral margin of cancer lesion, endoscopic clipping before surgery is performed. There are several modified techniques of LADG, but the most common techniques in LADG with D1 + α lymph node dissection consisted of the following procedures [3]:

(1) After CO_2 pneumoperitoneum is created, the four trocars are placed at the upper abdomen.

(2) Under laparoscopic procedures, the greater and lesser omentums and the gastrocolic ligament are dissected.

(3) The right gastroepiploric vessels are cut to dissect the subpyloric lymph nodes (number 6).

(4) The suprapyloric lymph nodes are dissected after cutting of the right gastric artery (number 5).

(5) The left gastric vessels are divided, and the left cardiac and superior gastric lymph nodes are dissected (numbers 1, 3, 7).

(6) After mobilization of the stomach and D1 + α lymph node dissection under laparoscopic procedures, a 5-cm laparotomy is made below the xyphoid.

(7) The duodenum and the distal portion of the stomach are exteriorized through this minilaparotomy.

(8) The distal gastrectomy with D1 + α lymph nodes is performed with a linear stapler.

(9) Usually, the reconstruction by Billroth-I method is performed.

Present status of laparoscopy-assisted distal gastrectomy

There are three types of laparoscopic gastrectomy: the totally laparoscopic procedure, the laparoscopy-assisted procedure, and the hand-assisted laparoscopic procedure. The laparoscopy-assisted procedure is the most popular because the resected specimen can be pulled out of the abdominal cavity through the small laparotomy incision.

Laparoscopic distal, proximal, and total gastrectomy are performed according to the location of the tumor and depth of invasion, as in open surgery. In Asian countries, LADG is the most frequently used procedure. In Japan, the JSES survey showed that 2600 patients underwent LADG for gastric cancer during the period 1991 to 2001 [15]. Pylorus-preserving gastrectomy and vagus-preserving gastrectomy techniques have recently been developed for early gastric cancer.

Because laparoscopic gastrectomy was developed as a treatment for early gastric cancer, it is most often performed with D1 + α lymph node dissection. According to the JSES survey [15], D1 + α lymph node dissection was performed in 67% and D2 lymph node dissection in 23% of LADGs in Japan.

Evaluation of laparoscopy-assisted distal gastrectomy

The results of LADG have been investigated since 1995. There have been several case-controlled studies comparing LADG with open gastrectomy, and a few randomized controlled studies on the short-term outcome of LADG (Table 3). We have seven studies about outcome and evaluation of LADG to date. All studies, showed some advantages, including early recovery, less pain, and less invasiveness in LADG.

Table 3
Evaluation of LADG for cancer

First author	Report	Cases (LADG/DG)	Advantage of LADG
Short-term clinical outcome			
Kitano S	Surg (2002) [26]	14/14 (RCT)	Less pain, less impaired pulmonary function
Adachi Y	Arch Surg (2000) [27]	49/53 (case)	Less surgical trauma, less impaired nutrition
Yano H	Gastric Cancer (2001) [28]	24/35 (case)	Less pain, shorter hospital stay
			Shorter times to the first passing of flatus, first walking, restarting of oral intake
			Shorter hospital stay, less pain
Reyes CD	Surg Endosc (2001) [29]	18/18 (case)	Earlier return to bowel function, shorter hospital stay
Mochiki E	World J Surg (2002) [30]	24/31 (case)	Shorter hospital stay, rapid recovery of bowel function
			Lower rate of postoperative complication
Migoh S	Hepato-gastro (2003) [31]	10/17 (case)	Earlier start of liquid diet, lower level of serum CRP
Weber KJ	Surg Endosc (2003) [32]	12/13 (case)	Earlier return to bowel function, shorter hospital stay
Immunofunction			
Fujii K	Surg Endosc (2003) [33]	10/10 (case)	Preservation of postoperative Th1 cell function
Cost			
Adachi Y	Surg Endosc (2001) [34]	48/43 (case)	Less expensive
Patient's QOL (questionnaire)			
Adachi Y	Ann Surg (1999) [35]	41/35 (case)	Better patient
Goh PMY	Surg Endosc (1997) [36]	16 surgeons	Superior to the open techniques (10 of 16 surgeons)

Abbreviation: QOL, quality of life.

There are currently no adequate data to determine the long-term outcome of LADG.

Short-term outcome
Operative findings. Reports of operation time for LADG differ. Mochiki et al [30] reported a longer operation time for LADG than for open distal gastrectomy (DG) (199.8 versus 238 minutes, $P = 0.002$). In contrast, Adachi and coauthors [27] and Yano and colleagues [28] reported no significant difference in operation time between the procedures. The operation time seems to depend on the learning curve of the surgical team; however, most studies found significantly decreased blood loss with LADG in comparison to DG. This may result from the use of laparoscopic coagulating shears under the amplified operative field in LADG.

There have been several comparative studies of morbidity associated with LADG and DG. Adachi and coworkers [27] reported the same rate of complications with LADG as with DG; however, Mochiki and associates [30] found that postoperative ileus was less frequent with LADG than with DG (2% versus 19%, $P = 0.003$). Yano et al [28] showed that the morbidity rate with LADG was lower than with DG (4.2% versus 11.4%, $P < 0.05$). In addition, there have been a few reports about outcomes in case series. Asao and colleagues [37] reported no serious complications in their series. Fujiwara and coauthors [38] warned of a high incidence (14%) of anastomotic leakage with LADG, despite the use of a circular stapler.

According to the JSES survey, the morbidity and mortality associated with LADG were 9.7% and 0%, respectively. These results suggest that LADG is a safe procedure.

Histological findings in resected specimens. The curability of LADG is discussed in terms of the resected margin and the number of dissected lymph nodes. Weber et al [32] reported that all resected margins were free of tumor in 12 laparoscopic surgery cases. Adachi and colleagues [27] indicated that the proximal margin of resected specimens was the same with LADG as DG (6.2 versus 6.0 cm).

Most comparative studies of the number of dissected lymph nodes found no significant difference between LADG with D1 + α and DG with D1 + α lymph node dissection. Furthermore, Miura et al [39] showed that LADG with D2 resection yielded a sufficient number of nodes for adequate TNM classification (> 15 nodes) in 86% of patients, suggesting that LADG may be appropriate for more advanced cancer. Thus, the histological findings indicate that LADG is as much curative procedure for early gastric cancer as open gastrectomy.

Postoperative course. It is difficult to assess the effect of reduced invasiveness of LADG on the postoperative course, because there is no objective measure. Many reports, however, confirm that the less invasive procedure, in comparison to open surgery, is associated with rapid return of gastrointestinal function, shorter hospital stay, and less pain. In a randomized controlled trial, Kitano and associates [26] identified several advantages of LADG, including lower Visual Analog Scale (VAS) pain score and decreased impairment of pulmonary function as determined by Forced Vital Capacity (FVC) and Forced Expiratory Volume in 1 Second (FEV1). In a case-controlled study, Adachi and colleagues [27] found decreased leukocyte counts on days 1 and 3, decreased granulocyte counts on day 1, and decreased levels of serum of C-reactive protein (CRP), interleukin-6, and albumin on day 1 or 3. Furthermore, weight loss with LADG was less than that with Distal Gastrectomy (DG), suggesting reduced nutritional impairment after LADG. Migoh and coworkers [31] also observed a lower serum CRP level on postoperative day 3 with LADG (4.2 versus 9.4, $P < 0.05$). Fujii et al [31] examined the immune responses after LADG, and found that LADG contributed to the preservation of postsurgical Th1 cell-mediated immune function. Goh and coauthors [36] surveyed surgeons worldwide, and found that laparoscopic gastrectomy was considered superior to open surgery by 10 of 16 surgeons because of faster recovery, less pain, and better cosmesis. In another questionnaires-based study, Adachi and colleagues [35] found that patients reported a better postoperative QOL after LADG than after DG.

Thus, to the extent that postoperative course reflects the effect of surgical invasion, the reduced invasiveness of LADG appears beneficial.

Cost. There has been only one study on the cost of LADG [34]. According to this study, LADG is less expensive than DG because both the postoperative recovery period and hospital stay are shorter.

Long-term outcome

There have been few reports on the long-term outcome of LADG for early gastric cancer. Kitano et al [40] successfully performed 116 LADGs for early gastric cancer over 10 years, and all patients except one, who died not of cancer but of cerebral bleeding, were alive without recurrence or port-site metastasis during a mean follow-up period of 45 months. Randomized controlled trials and case-controlled studies to compare long-term survival after LADG are warranted.

Laparoscopic surgery for other tumors

Surgeons have begun to use laparoscopic procedures to treat tumors other than early gastric cancer. These include GIST and malignant lymphoma.

Laparoscopic surgery for gastric gastrointestinal submucosal tumor

Indications

Leiomyoma or leiomyosarcoma is the most common type of GIST in the stomach. Leiomyosarcoma of the stomach represents about 1% to 3% of primary malignant tumors and about 20% of submucosal tumors of the stomach [41]. If lymph node dissection is necessary for surgical management of gastric leiomyosarcoma, total gastrectomy is often required because about 60% of leiomyosarcomas are located in the upper third of the stomach. Lindsay et al [42], however, reported that in a group of 50 patients, none had lymph node metastasis, suggesting that lymph node dissection was not necessary. Thus, there are few reports in which the presence of lymph node metastasis in leiomyosarcoma measuring less than 5 cm in diameter is described. Estes and associates [43] recommended wedge resection of the stomach with a tumor-free margin for the treatment of leiomyosarcoma. Also, Yoshida and coauthors [44] concluded from a retrospective study that LWR can be considered the first-line treatment for gastric leiomyosarcoma.

Present status of laparoscopic wedge resection

There are several case reports of LWR for GIST. Bouillot and colleagues [45] reviewed 65 cases of gastric GIST in 20 centers in France, and Choi et al [46] reported 32 cases of gastric GIST treated by laparoscopic surgery. The JSES survey [15] showed that in Japan, 629 cases of gastric GIST were treated with LWR and 475 with laparoscopic gastrectomy during the period 1991 to 2001; the morbidity rate was 3.2%. In Japan, a large leiomyoma is considered an indication for laparoscopic gastrectomy with lymph node dissection.

The evaluation of laparoscopic wedge resection

Although many cases of LWR for gastric GIST have been reported, only one retrospective study comparing short-term outcomes of LWR versus open wedge resection has been performed [47]. According to this study, LWR for gastric GIST has several advantages, including earlier oral intake, shorter hospital stay, and reduced use of analgesics, despite the longer operation time. Although there are not a sufficient number of studies to evaluate the short- and long-term outcomes of LWR, LWR seems to be a feasible treatment for gastric GIST.

Laparoscopic surgery for other tumors

There have been several case reports of laparoscopic surgery for other types of tumors, including nonepithelial and submucosal tumor. Yasuda and coauthors [5] applied LADG to treat a malignant lymphoma of the stomach, and Benitez et al [48] performed LWR for B-cell gastric mucosa-associated lymphoid tissue lymphoma. Harold and colleagues [49] reported using LWR for symptomatic pancreatic rests located in the stomach.

Summary

Since 1991, laparoscopic surgery has been used to treat gastric tumors, including gastric cancer and gastric GIST. Although laparoscopic gastric resection for gastric tumors has not been accepted worldwide, its use has rapidly increased in Asian countries because of earlier recovery, earlier hospital discharge, less pain, and good cosmesis without a decrease in operative curability. To establish laparoscopic surgery as a standard treatment for gastric tumors, multicenter randomized controlled clinical trials are needed to compare the short- and long-term outcomes of laparoscopic versus open means of access.

References

[1] McMahon AJ, Russell IT, Ramsay G, et al. Laparoscopic and minilaparotomy cholecystectomy: a randomized trial comparing postoperative pain and pulmonary function. Surgery 1994;115:533–9.
[2] Redmond HP, Watson RW, Houghton T, et al. Immune function in patients undergoing open vs laparoscopic cholecystectomy. Arch Surg 1994;129:1240–6.
[3] Kitano S, Iso Y, Moriyama M, et al. Laparoscopy-assisted Billroth I gastrectomy. Surg Laparosc Endosc 1994;4:146–8.
[4] Ohgami M, Otani Y, Furukawa T, et al. Curative laparoscopic surgery for early gastric cancer: eight years experience. Nippon Geka Gakkai Zasshi 2000;101:539–45.
[5] Yasuda K, Shiraishi N, Adachi Y, et al. Laparoscopy-assisted distal gastrectomy for malignant lymphoma. Surg Laparosc Endosc Percutan Tech 2001;11:372–4.
[6] Watson DI, Devitt PG, Game PA. Laparoscopic Billroth II gastrectomy for early gastric cancer. Br J Surg 1995;82:661–2.
[7] Uyama I, Ogiwara H, Takahara T, et al. Laparoscopic and minilaparotomy proximal gastrectomy and esophagogastrostomy: technique and case report. Surg Endosc 1995;5: 487–91.
[8] Taniguchi S, Koga K, Ibusuki K, et al. Laparoscopic pylorus-preserving gastrectomy with intracorporeal hand-sewn anastomosis. Surg Endosc Laparosc 1997;7:354–6.
[9] Uyama I, Sugioka A, Fujita J, et al. Complete laparoscopic extraperigastric lymph node dissection for gastric malignancies located in the middle or lower third of the stomach. Gastric Cancer 1999;2:186–90.
[10] Ohki J, Nagai H, Hyodo M, et al. Hand-assisted laparoscopic distal gastrectomy with abdominal wall-lifting method. Surg Endosc 1999;13:1148–50.
[11] Kitano S, Adachi Y, Shiraishi N, et al. Laparoscopic-assisted proximal gastrectomy for early gastric carcinomas. Surg Today 1999;29:389–91.
[12] Goh PM, Khan AZ, So JB, et al. Early experience with laparoscopic radical gastrectomy for advanced gastric cancer. Surg Laparosc Endosc Percutan Tech 2001;11:83–7.
[13] Uyama I, Sugioka A, Matsui H, et al. Laparoscopic side-to-side esophagogastrostomy using a linear stapler after proximal gastrectomy. Gastric Cancer 2001;4:98–102.
[14] Mochiki E, Kamimura H, Haga N, et al. The technique of laparoscopically assisted total gastrectomy with jejunal interposition for early gastric cancer. Surg Endosc 2001;16:540–4.
[15] Japan Society for Endoscopic Surgery. Nationwide survey on endoscopic surgery in Japan. Journal of Japan Society Endoscopic Surgery 2002;7:479–567 [in Japanese].
[16] Ohashi S. Laparoscopic intraluminal (intragastric) surgery for early gastric cancer. Surg Endosc 1995;9:169–71.
[17] Hyung WJ, Cheong JH, Kim J, et al. Application of minimally invasive treatment for early gastric cancer. J Surg Oncol 2004;85:181–5.

[18] Japanese Gastric Cancer Association. The guidelines for the treatment of gastric cancer. Tokyo: Kachara Co. 2001.

[19] Ono H, Kondo H, Gotoda T, et al. Endoscopic mucosal resection for treatment of early gastric cancer. Gut 2001;48:225–9.

[20] Kitagawa Y, Ohgami M, Fujii H, et al. Laparoscopic detection of sentinel lymph nodes in gastrointestinal cancer: a novel and minimally invasive approach. Ann Surg Oncol 2001;8: 86–9.

[21] Shimizu S, Noshiro H, Nagai E, et al. Laparoscopic gastric surgery in a Japanese institution: analysis of the initial 100 procedures. J Am Coll Surg 2003;197:372–8.

[22] Kobayashi T, Kazui T, Kimura T. Surgical local resection for early gastric cancer. Surg Laparosc Endosc Percutan Tech 2003;13:299–303.

[23] Omote K, Mai M, Mizoguchi M, et al. Degree of submucosal invasion of early carcinoma and risk for lymph node metastasis: consideration limiting of applicability for endoscopic resection (in Japanese, with abstract in English). Stomach Intest 1997;32:49–55.

[24] Oizumi H, Matsuda T, Fukase K, et al. Endoscopic resection for early gastric cancer: the actual procedure and clinical evaluation (in Japanese, with abstract in English). Stomach Intest 1991;26:289–300.

[25] Fujii K, Okajima K, Isozaki H, et al. A clinicopathological study on the indications of limited surgery for submucosal gastric cancer (in Japanese, with abstract in English). Jpn J Gastroenterol Surg 1998;31:2055–62.

[26] Kitano S, Shiraishi N, Fujii K, et al. A randomized controlled trial comparing open vs laparoscopy-assisted distal gastrectomy for the treatment of early gastric cancer: an interim report. Surgery 2002;131:S306–11.

[27] Adachi Y, Shiraishi N, Shiromizu A, et al. Laparoscopy-assisted Billroth I gastrectomy compared with conventional open gastrectomy. Arch Surg 2000;135:806–10.

[28] Yano H, Monden T, Kinuta M, et al. The usefulness of laparoscopy-assisted distal gastrectomy in comparison with that of open distal gastrectomy for early gastric cancer. Gastric Cancer 2001;4:93–7.

[29] Reyes CD, Weber KJ, Gagner M, et al. Laparoscopic vs open gastrectomy. A retrospective review. Surg Endosc 2001;15:928–31.

[30] Mochiki E, Nakabayashi T, Kamimura H, et al. Gastrointestinal recovery and outcome after laparoscopy-assisted versus conventional open distal gastrectomy for early gastric cancer. World J Surg 2002;26:1145–9.

[31] Migoh S, Hasuda K, Nakashima K, et al. The benefit of laparoscopy-assisted distal gastrectomy compared with conventional open distal gastrectomy: a case-matched control study. Hepatogastroenterology 2003;50:2251–4.

[32] Weber KJ, Reyes CD, Gagner M, et al. Comparison of laparoscopic and open gastrectomy for malignant disease. Surg Endosc 2003;17:968–71.

[33] Fujii K, Sonoda K, Izumi K, et al. T lymphocyte subsets and Th1/Th2 balance after laparoscopy-assisted distal gastrectomy. Surg Endosc 2003;17:1440–4.

[34] Adachi Y, Shiraishi N, Ikebe K, et al. Evaluation of the cost for laparoscopic-assisted Billroth I gastrectomy. Surg Endosc 2001;15:932–6.

[35] Adachi Y, Suematsu T, Shiraishi N, et al. Quality of life after laparoscopy-assisted Billroth I gastrectomy. Ann Surg 1999;229:49–54.

[36] Goh PMY, Alponat A, Mak K, et al. Early international results of laparoscopic gastrectomies. Surg Endosc 1997;11:650–2.

[37] Asao T, Hosouchi Y, Nakabayashi T, et al. Laparoscopically assisted or distal gastrectomy with lymph node dissection for early gastric cancer. Br J Surg 2001;88:128–32.

[38] Fujiwara M, Kodera Y, Kasai Y, et al. Laparoscopy-assisted distal gastrectomy with systemic lymph node dissection for early gastric carcinoma: a review of 43 cases. J Am Coll Surg 2003;196:75–81.

[39] Miura S, Kodera Y, Fujiwara M, et al. Laparoscopy-assisted distal gastrectomy with systemic lymph node dissection: a critical reappraisal from the viewpoint of lymph node retrieval. J Am Coll Surg 2004;198:933–8.

[40] Kitano S, Shiraishi N, Kakisako K, et al. Laparoscopy-assisted Billroth-I gastrectomy (LADG) for cancer: our 10 years' experience. Surg Laparosc Endosc Percutan Tech 2002;12: 204–7.

[41] Bandoh T, Isoyama T, Toyoshima H. Submucosal tumors of the stomach: a study of 100 operative cases. Surgery 1993;13:498–506.

[42] Lindsay PC, Ordonez N, Raaf JH. Gastric leiomyosarcoma: clinical and pathological review of fifty patients. J Surg Oncol 1981;18:399–421.

[43] Estes NC, Cherian G, Haller CC. Advanced gastric leiomyosarcoma. Am Surg 1989;55: 353–5.

[44] Yoshida M, Otani Y, Ohgami M, et al. Surgical management of gastric leiomyosarcoma: evaluation of the propriety of laparoscopic wedge resection. World J Surg 1997;21:440–3.

[45] Bouillot JL, Bresler L, Fragniez PL, et al. Laparoscopic resection of benign submucosal stomach tumors. A report of 65 cases. Gastroenterol Clin Biol 2003;27:272–6.

[46] Choi YB, Oh ST. Laparoscopy in the management of gastric submucosal tumors. Surg Endosc 2000;14:741–5.

[47] Cheng HL, Lee WJ, Lai IR, et al. Laparoscopic wedge resection of benign gastric tumor. Hepatogastroenterology 1999;46:2100–4.

[48] Benitez LD, Edelman DS. Gastroscopic-assisted laparoscopic wedge resection of B-cell gastric mucosa-associated lymphoid tissue (MALT) lymphoma. Surg Endosc 1999;13:62–4.

[49] Harold KL, Sturdevant M, Matthews BD, et al. Ectopic pancreatic tissue presenting as submucosal gastric mass. J Laparoendosc Adv Surg Tech A 2002;12:333–8.

ELSEVIER
SAUNDERS

Surg Clin N Am 85 (2005) 165–168

SURGICAL
CLINICS OF
NORTH AMERICA

Index

Note: Page numbers of article titles are in **boldface** type.

Changing Your Address?

Make sure your subscription changes too! When you notify us of your new address, you can help make our job easier by including an exact copy of your Clinics label number with your old address (see illustration below.) This number identifies you to our computer system and will speed the processing of your address change. Please be sure this label number accompanies your old address and your corrected address—you can send an old Clinics label with your number on it or just copy it exactly and send it to the address listed below.

We appreciate your help in our attempt to give you continuous coverage. Thank you.

W. B. Saunders Company

SHIPPING AND RECEIVING DEPTS.
151 BENIGNO BLVD.
BELLMAWR, N.J. 08031

SECOND CLASS POSTAGE
PAID AT BELLMAWR, N.J.

This is your copy of the
_____ CLINICS OF NORTH AMERICA

00503570 DOE—J32400   101   NH   8102

JOHN C DOE MD
324 SAMSON ST
BERLIN   NH   03570

XP-D11494

JAN ISSUE

Your Clinics Label Number

Copy it exactly or send your label along with your address to:
W.B. Saunders Company, Customer Service
Orlando, FL 32887-4800
Call Toll Free 1-800-654-2452

Please allow four to six weeks for delivery of new subscriptions and for processing address changes.

BUSINESS REPLY MAIL

FIRST-CLASS MAIL   PERMIT NO 7135   ORLANDO FL

POSTAGE WILL BE PAID BY ADDRESSEE

PERIODICALS ORDER FULFILLMENT DEPT
ELSEVIER
6277 SEA HARBOR DR
ORLANDO FL 32821-9816